Also by George Beddingfield

Hush, Boy
Conditional
Unannounced

WILDFIRE

George Beddingfield

WILDFIRE is a work of fiction. All names, characters, and incidents are creations of the author's imagination or they are used fictiously. Any resemblance to actual persons, living or dead, is entirely coincidental

ISBN-13: 978-1500918033
ISBN-10: 1500918032
Library of Congress Control Number: 2014915406
CreateSpace Independent Publishing Platform, North Charleston, SC

DEDICATION

For all the men and women on all of Earth's continents who live with the human immunodeficiency virus. Until very recently medical science had never produced a cure for a viral disease, and that one is not yet proved. For some a successful vaccine has emerged, but never a proven cure. Keep alive the hope that this virus will be the next to be eradicated by a cure.

ACKNOWLEDGMENTS

Over the years a few friends have unknowingly shown me what it's like to live with HIV positive status. Some have fallen victim to AIDS, and their experiences have saddened me. Others enjoy near-normal lives, and I rejoice with them. I am grateful for all I've learned from every one of them.

Communications and publications of amfAR, the American Foundation for AIDS Research, most recently its countdown to a cure by 2020, have reassured me that hope is alive. Many thanks to amfAR for excellent work.

My years at Tulane University and the New Orleans Charity Hospital have provided the rich background of a fascinating region that became the setting for this novel. I am grateful for those fine years of opportunity and challenge.

Roxie Montesano's unstinting loyalty and his helpful critiques as the first reader for each of my chapters have been invaluable. Special thanks to Roxie for continuing to tolerate my need for solitary writing time.

George Beddingfield
August 2014

1

INFECTED

AROUND ELEVEN O'CLOCK ON A WARM AUGUST NIGHT IN 1987, Jeremy Becker stood at Doug's bedside in a dimly lighted New Orleans hospital ward. Without air conditioning humidity was high. Nearby patients slept beneath light sheets or none at all. Human smells of sick men overrode the ward's undertones of antiseptic solutions and cleaning fluids. Night lights threw menacing shadows onto the ceiling .

Jeremy was a medical student and he'd learned scut work was part of the deal, even late night scut work. He turned on his flashlight, then touched Doug's shoulder and shook him gently. Doug didn't respond at all. Fever's got him disoriented, Jeremy thought. No problem. Doug didn't need an explanation anyway, not after more than twenty years of multiple transfusions and frequent blood drawing—lifelong treatment for hemophilia. Jeremy decided he could probably do what he had to do without even waking his patient, so he tightened a rubber tourniquet around Doug's upper arm.

He pulled off his hospital coat and tossed it across the foot of the bed, then rolled his shirt sleeves up to his elbows and finger combed his short blond hair off his forehead. He poked at the inside of Doug's elbow until his probing fingers felt a vein just below the tourniquet. He knew Doug wouldn't hear him, but he spoke to him anyway as he pulled on a pair of latex gloves, then swabbed the area with an alcohol sponge and pulled the skin taut. "This'll only take a couple of seconds then you can go back to sleep, okay? Here comes the needle stick." He slid the needle through Doug's skin and guided it into the vein. Blood flowed into the collection tube.

Confused, Doug jerked away hard. "No, doc, please don't do it. No more transfusions. Come on, not tonight."

In that instant of lost control the bloody needle twisted out of Doug's arm and plunged into the back of Jeremy's own hand—pierced the latex glove and stabbed deep into the space between his left thumb and index finger.

"Goddamn it!" Jeremy yelled. He yanked the needle out of his hand and, in a flash of anger, he almost punched the patient. Doug was quiet, completely unaware of the accident. Jeremy relaxed, then shook his head and released the tourniquet. Doug had already developed a large purple bruise beneath the skin, and blood oozed from the puncture site. Jeremy wiped the blood away from his patient's arm and pressed a gauze pad over the purple spot—pressed firmly until he noticed a growing circle of blood inside the glove on his own left hand.

Turning to the sink, he stripped off his gloves and squeezed a drop of blood from the tiny puncture near the base of his thumb. The wound looked insignificant, but Jeremy knew it could be more. He scrubbed his hands with soap and water, scrubbed a second time, then wiped the harmless looking puncture wound with alcohol and put a Band-Aid over it.

Shitty luck, he thought. This bastard's HIV-positive. Who was that woman that got AIDS from a needle stick five or six years ago? Baltimore? No, New York. Italian sounding name. Prego—something like that. Wonder what ever became of her. Probably died of AIDS.

Christ, could that happen to him? No way—that was rare. Still, maybe he should report the accident to his chief...but what the hell for? Too late now. The resident would put him through all that hospital rigmarole about needle punctures anyway—plenty of time for reporting it later.

Jeremy looked down again at his sleeping patient—completely out of it like nothing had happened. Doug's hemophilia had required clotting factor transfusions before blood banks routinely tested donors for the Human Immunodeficiency Virus. One of those transfusions was later found to be HIV-positive. A few months afterward Doug's ELISA, a screening blood test for HIV, turned positive.

Curious in the early days of their relationship, Jeremy had asked, "How'd you react, Doug? How'd you feel when you found out you'd tested positive?"

"Mad at first," Doug had said. "Yeah, I was mad as hell 'cause it happened to me. It took a while, but I managed to work through all that 'why me' shit." He got quiet after that, volunteered nothing more.

Jeremy hesitated. He hadn't intended to bring up painful memories for his new patient, but he wanted to know what it was like to have the HIV time bomb in your body, felt he needed to know it as a physician-to-be. "Looks like you've handled it pretty well—going to grad school and all."

Doug nodded. "Yeah, I'm okay now, but it was real tough at first." He pared a fleck of brown clay from beneath a fingernail. "Look, I know the damn virus causes AIDS, but so far I've been lucky. No sign of AIDS. I'm countin' on somebody discoverin' a cure before I progress that far." He grinned. "Maybe you'll be the one who finds the cure, Dr. Becker."

"Listen, don't call me doctor. You know I'm a medical student—besides, we're just about the same age."

"I know. But I've been around hospitals most of my life. I know the rules. Anyway, you're practically a doctor. What is it, anyway—another year and a half of the rat race?"

"About that," Jeremy said. "A year from next June."

"It really takes guts to go to med school—I've seen the hard work and long hours. I admire you guys, Dr. Becker."

"Thanks, but I meant what I said…just call me Jeremy." He closed the cover of Doug's medical chart, then smiled. "You can call me Dr. Becker if I get accepted for the surgery residency."

"Surgery? You really are ambitious—I hear that's a tough nut to crack."

"Right...but it's the only thing I've wanted since I started thinking about specialties. I just hope I get accepted for the residency."

"From what I see, they'll have a hard time keepin' you out."

Jeremy waved off that remark. "Thanks, Doug. That's nice to hear from a guy like you. You must work pretty hard yourself." He raised his eyebrows. "How much longer for you? About six months, is it, to finish your MFA? I'll bet you get a faculty appointment after that. I've seen your sculpture. It's good, Doug, real good."

"Come on, my work's not that big a deal…I just do what I like."

Jeremy smiled. He admired modesty in a real achiever. "How do you keep on pushing, Doug? How do you plan for the future when you know you're infected with HIV? Why don't you just quit? What keeps you from stoppin' everything you do and waitin' for AIDS to happen?"

"Oh, boy, that's the sixty-four dollar question. There were plenty of days when I wanted to do that…too many days." Doug pulled on a robe and tied the belt around his slim waist. "Listen, I know just about everybody that's HIV-positive develops AIDS sooner or later. And I know just about everybody with AIDS dies." He glanced at Jeremy. "The ones I've seen had a pretty bad time of it toward the end." He didn't speak for a while, just stood there and let his shoulders droop. Then he looked up and scratched his chin. "Enough of that crap, Doc. Let's just say I've made up my mind not to worry about things I can't do anything about."

Jeremy had admired that attitude from the first day he met Doug—he had refused to let his positive HIV blood test get in the way of his plans for the future. But now, months later, all that had changed. Doug's fever was soaring, and that could mean progression of his HIV disease. AIDS could be closing in on him.

Now this shit had happened to Jeremy. He'd long known chores like blood drawing were delegated to medical students at the New Orleans Charity Hospital, but, man, that damn needle stick was more than he'd bargained for. What the hell? No use worrying about that right now—it probably wouldn't amount to much anyway.

Rubbing the Band-Aid on his left hand, he walked to the opposite side of the bed to draw the blood from Doug's other arm. No difficulty that time. A few days later Doug's fever proved to be transfusion related and he left the hospital. No sign of HIV progression. At the end of November Jeremy completed his hematology assignment and rotated to another hospital unit.

Charity's protocol for needle stick accidents included a series of blood tests for HIV, even though incidents like that rarely caused infection. At first negative, Jeremy's ELISA converted to positive two months after the accident. A repeat ELISA was positive, and that meant his immune system was making antibodies in an effort to fight some virus.

The Western Blot, a more specific blood test for the AIDS virus, was also positive. The infection Jeremy's body was gearing up to fight was caused by the HIV, no doubt about that. The AIDS time bomb was living in his body and there wasn't a damn thing he could do about it. Acquired Immune Deficiency Syndrome became his own personal demon, something he'd worry about every day and every night for the rest of his life. Anti-retroviral treatment was just coming into its own in research circles. Shit, what about his dream of a surgery residency? What about his hope for years of work with patients who needed his skills in the operating room? What about his life?

2

World AIDS Day

During another late night session twenty-two years later Dr. Jeremy Becker pushed aside the papers and medical journals covering his desk. He pulled off his reading glasses and leaned back in his leather chair to mull over exactly what he should tell the physicians' group which had invited him to give the keynote address at an upcoming conference planned to begin on World AIDS Day. The invitation had come to him because he'd lived through the evolution of understanding about HIV infections, and he'd witnessed myriad advancements in treatment for HIV and AIDS. He'd lived through those things all right—lived through them on a very personal basis. He thought he should tell the conference about his life—what it was like before the virus, how things changed after he was infected.

The AIDS conference was a huge undertaking, planned for as a time to present the history of HIV infections in humans and the latest developments in AIDS treatment. Several thousand attendees were expected to crowd into the Louisiana Superdome for Jeremy's keynote address. World AIDS Day, observed on December 1 every year, was on a Thursday that year and the opening session would kick off a long weekend of scholarly presentations by physicians and researchers from around the world.

The idea for a special day to raise awareness of the worldwide AIDS pandemic was conceived by a team of information officers at the World Health Organization's Geneva headquarters and later adopted by the United Nations. All U.N. member states had observed World AIDS Days since 1988, and all of them had adopted the red ribbon as a symbol of support and solidarity for HIV-positive people and people living with AIDS.

Jeremy turned off his desk lamp and rubbed his eyes. He lifted his coffee mug to his lips, but the mug was empty—nothing left but the cold dregs of an earlier *café latte.* Not ready yet to call it a night, he left his study and headed for the kitchen. More coffee might help him figure out how to begin the speech.

He was surprised to find his wife at her desk in the kitchen. "Oh, hi, Barb. I didn't know you were still up. I'm gonna make another cup of coffee. Want one?"

"No thanks, but I will have a little brandy if you're pouring."

"Sure," Jeremy said. "What are you doing, anyway? I thought you'd be asleep by now."

"Nothing much—just planning a menu for our dinner party next month. I knew you were working on your keynote address, so I thought I'd just stay out of your way."

Nudging up behind her, Jeremy squeezed her shoulders and kissed the top of her head. "You know you could never get in my way. Anyhow, I want to talk to you—how do you think I should start the speech. I think I want to tell 'em how I got HIV and what it felt like to get that death sentence."

"Death sentence?" Barbara said. "What do you mean, death sentence? You've been living and doing pretty well for more than twenty years since that needle stick. Anyway, about your speech…I suppose the infectious disease experts are gonna tell the conference about how treatments have changed and all that."

"I'm sure they will, but what can a surgeon tell 'em? I'm supposed to get everybody charged up about how much the whole AIDS business has changed in recent times."

"Well there you are, Jere. Tell 'em about all that stuff we went through in the early nineties. Tell 'em how pleased they should be that some of those crazy things have changed. Tell 'em how HIV-positive folks can now live pretty normal lives…like us."

"You mean tell about all that segregation in the late 80s—the Health Protection Act and all that? Wouldn't they already know about that bad idea?"

"Listen, Jeremy, a lot of the people at the conference will be too young to have lived through those times like we did—and many of the others didn't know about it from their own personal experience. Tell 'em how it came about. Tell 'em everything about that stupid law. Tell 'em how personal greed got in the way and led to the end of the big research push"

"Good idea. That kind of background might set the pace for the whole conference. You've got me going now. I'll have to work on those ideas. Don't wait up for me, Barb. I have a feeling it's gonna be a long night."

Jeremy took his fresh *café latte* back to his study to tackle that approach to the opening of his keynote address. He'd tell 'em about those early days in the history of HIV as a worldwide health concern—tell it from the viewpoint of his own experience with the damn virus, tell about the fear-driven political reforms the spreading epidemic led to. He'd tell 'em the whole story. Just thinking about all of that opened a huge world of old memories for Jeremy, some of them good memories, others not so good.

3

A New Law

EARLY ON A SPRING MORNING, YEARS BEFORE HIS ALL-NIGHT work on the keynote address, a premonition had hit Jeremy as soon as he stretched his lean body out of bed. He had a feeling of expectancy, an undefined dread, like something really bad was about to happen. Walking toward the full length bedroom window, he slowed down to check his reflection in the dresser mirror. Looked like his weight was holding. Not bad, actually, considering he hadn't worked out in a couple of weeks because of finals.

He'd had the garage apartment on Henry Clay Avenue through four years of medical school, a lucky break that came his way because the owner who'd renovated the place was a former classmate of his father. In earlier days, when the estate was in its heyday, the garage apartment had been the coachman's quarters over a carriage house. For Jeremy it had provided the quiet and privacy he needed to master the vast amount of information from his medical classes. He had spent long hours studying there until now, at long last, that part of his life was about to end…he would soon become Jeremy Becker, M.D.

The morning was shaping up to become one of those rare days in New Orleans when the air was both cool and dry and nobody had to use air conditioning. Standing at the open window, Jeremy inhaled the fragrances of garden loam and new-mown grass—the fresh smells of spring. Blinking in the hazy morning light, he gazed out across the hedges that separated the driveway from an expanse of lush green turf with scattered azaleas and other flowering shrubs. He spotted Dr. Abingdon, his landlord, sitting at a wrought iron table on the patio behind the main house.

Abingdon looked up, then waved toward the window and held up a cup. "Morning, Jeremy. Join me for coffee." Then, with a sarcastic twist to his words, he said, "Let's celebrate the big day."

Jeremy knew exactly what was bothering Dr. Abingdon. At first blush the new law had troubled him, too, but he'd decided he could go along with most of it. At least he'd know what to count on when he became a surgeon—and he was set on that. Ignoring Abingdon's sarcasm, he grinned and returned the wave. "Thanks—be right down."

"Uh...Jeremy."

"Yes, sir?"

"You'd better put on some clothes first. Marian's here."

Jeremy realized, then, he was standing naked at the tall window, probably visible, even though the screen. He laughed and covered himself with the curtain. "Sorry about that. Be down in a minute."

When Jeremy reached the patio, Dr. Abingdon took a fresh cup and poured strong black coffee with chicory from a pewter pot while pouring warm milk from another. Good, Jeremy thought, *café au lait*. The rich, savory aroma of New Orleans coffee hit him even before he sat down. He noticed a basket of croissants, too, and his stomach growled. "Hey, this looks like a real celebration. I thought you were joking."

Abingdon scowled and shook his head. "You know better than that—I'm not celebrating anything. Marian just thought I deserved something nice on a rotten day like today." He grabbed up the front section of his morning paper and waved it in Jeremy's face. "Look at this garbage in *The Times-Picayune*. They've given this crap the whole front page. And that's not the worst of it—wait 'til you see the editorials."

So, he'd been right about Abingdon. Jeremy didn't think his landlord would be celebrating—not today. He glanced at the prominent page one headline: **HIV Law Begins Today**. "Well, people do need to know about the new regulations, Dr. Abingdon."

"Damn the regulations! We can't practice medicine like this." He jerked the paper open to the editorial page and shook it at Jeremy. "Just listen to this goddamn editor." Abingdon adjusted his half-frame glasses then shook his head and read, "Health Law Segregates HIV Carriers." He stopped and shook his head again. "This redneck editor thinks some kind of segregation's the answer to—"

"Don't let it upset you. He's just—"

"Don't interrupt me, Jeremy." He crushed the pages together, then laid the paper down and straightened his glasses once more before picking it up again. "Listen to this bullshit headline story: 'The Health Protection Act of 1989 becomes the law of the land today. This far-reaching piece of legislation is expected to do more than….' Where is that stupid part?"

Jeremy watched Abingdon scan down the page.

"Here it is. Listen. 'The new law requires every citizen to have a screening blood test for HIV. Confirmed positive tests will identify a person as HIV-positive, infected with the virus and capable of infecting others.'"

"Surely you knew—"

"Of course I knew, Jeremy. But this writer's holier-than-thou attitude is more than I can stomach. He likes all this regulation. Listen to this part. 'The law requires an HIV identity card for every person, and it includes measures to control and police every social opportunity for transmission of the lethal HIV. Every singles bar, gay bar, hotel and motel—every health club, blood bank, hospital, clinic and medical office—even every public toilet, will have its entry monitored by automated machines which require insertion of a person's HIV card and positive confirmation of identity. Entry will be denied to those whose HIV status differs from the building's designation.'"

"Nothing new there. We knew that was coming."

Abingdon slammed the newspaper down on the table. "The bastards are destroying America. What about freedom? What about civil liberties?"

"People are afraid, Dr. Abingdon. You know that."

Abingdon took off his reading glasses and checked his cup. "I know, I know.... Listen, don't pay any attention to me. I just like to bitch and moan—too old to change my ways, I guess." He shook his head and pushed the basket of croissants toward Jeremy. "Try those fig preserves. Marian's father made 'em."

He raised his eyebrows and looked Jeremy square in the eye. "Sounds like you're ready for this new law. You can't really like it, Jeremy. You're just going along, aren't you? Trying to be pragmatic about it?"

Jeremy knew he'd get on thin ice in a hurry in this conversation. He'd figured out from talking to his father that most older doctors weren't too happy about the Health Protection Act. "I admit the segregation's gonna take a little getting used to. From what I've learned, though, it might even be an improvement."

"Improvement? How in the hell can you say that?" Abingdon picked up the front section of the newspaper and folded it. "I thought I liked the *Picayune's* editor, but he makes it sound like the damn politicians have saved mankind from the medical profession. Does he really think we're a bunch of bumbling idiots?"

"I doubt if he believes that. Anyway—"

"I certainly hope not. He acted a lot smarter than that when I took care of his wife in the hospital last year."

Jeremy picked up another croissant and spooned fig preserves onto it. He worked at acting nonchalant, trying to stay flexible about the new law. He had to live with it, like it or not. "We had a special jurisprudence course on the Health Protection Act last semester. It's pretty complicated."

"How well I know that—I went to the medical society seminars about the damn thing. But they've gone too far, Jeremy." Abingdon shook his head as he poured more coffee for both of them. "I agree something had to be done, but this? The best I can say for it is now all the states will have the same laws at least."

"That's what I mean, Dr. Abingdon. That's the big improvement. Dad told me a few states passed some really crazy laws in the last few years." Jeremy stirred sugar into his coffee. "He said the medical societies fought the changes, but they couldn't do anything. The politicians wouldn't budge. Think about it. Doctors required to test themselves for HIV and inform their patients of the result, that kind of thing. Without this new law, that kind of stuff could wipe out a practice—could close it down completely. Surgeons couldn't even operate, bad things like that."

Abingdon nodded. "Your dad's right...how is he anyway? Will he be here for your graduation?"

"Dad's fine, busy as ever. Yeah, they're coming for graduation, but Mom's raising hell because she can't get him out of the office for more than three days. She wanted to make it a real vacation, but Dad says three days is long enough."

Abingdon smiled. "They're driving over?"

Jeremy nodded. His father, also a Tulane medical graduate, had taken his wife and young son to the east Texas city of Beaumont some twenty-five years earlier. Over the years his family practice had thrived and a great many East Texans had come to respect "Doc" Becker as the special guardian of their health care.

"Don't underestimate your dad," Abingdon said, "he's a good doctor. Let's all have dinner while they're here. I'll ask Marian to plan something special." He glanced at the newspaper laying on the table. "What else has he told you—what else about the state laws, I mean."

Jeremy shrugged. "More of the same. He said HIV-positive doctors couldn't do very much in a lot of states. Nurses either. No surgery. No invasive exams. Yet not one single state would allow doctors to require their patients to have an HIV test."

"That's true," Abingdon said, brushing crumbs from his tie. "They didn't worry much about preventing virus transfer from patients to doctors. Nobody wants to hear about that part of the problem."

"Some of us do," Jeremy said, with a wry smile. "I've been pretty interested in that part of it." Jeremy had told Dr. Abingdon he was HIV-positive. He'd told him about that needle stick accident while he was drawing blood from his hemophiliac patient who'd contracted HIV from a blood transfusion. He'd shared the bad news when his own HIV blood test converted to positive three months after the accident, and he'd kept him up to date on the complex medication regime he'd been on since that time.

Abingdon reached over and put a hand on Jeremy's shoulder. "How long, now, since that accident?"

"A little less than two years." Jeremy said. He'd grown accustomed to being HIV-positive—reached an accommodation with it for outward appearances anyway.

"I know it's been tough for you." Abingdon looked toward the garage apartment's window and chuckled. "But from the looks of things, I'd say you've done a pretty good job of taking care of yourself."

Jeremy shrugged. "I try. Oh, I feel great—no problem there. But, you know, I can never get away from it. I can never forget about the damn virus in my body. Staying busy helps, but the specter of AIDS never really goes away."

Abingdon shook his head. "Damn shame…whatever became of that patient who infected you?"

Jeremy put his cup down. "He died about four months ago—last January it was. Atypical pneumonia. He'd developed full-blown AIDS about a year after my needle stick. Tough break for a nice guy, brand new faculty appointment and all. He had a young wife, too."

"I'm sorry, Jeremy. I didn't know all that. Why didn't you tell me about it?"

"What could you do? Anyway, I'm fine so far." He drank the last of his coffee, then grinned. "Looks like the new law means I can take my surgery residency at Charity like I wanted. That makes up for a lot of the bad stuff."

Abingdon laughed. "Still call it Charity don't you?"

"Medical Center of Louisiana. The state can name it whatever they like—that grand old place will always be Big Charity to people who love it."

"I agree. And it's still one of the finest surgery programs in the country." Abingdon picked up the folded newspaper. "I'm glad to know something good will come from segregating the hospitals." He shook his head again. "How in God's name can they make buildings HIV-positive and negative? How in the hell can we practice medicine in that kind of world?"

"We can do it," Jeremy said. "You'll see."

❖❖❖

4

A New World

DR. ABINGDON PUT HIS CUP ON THE WROUGHT IRON TABLE and glanced at his watch. "I have to get moving, Jeremy. Here, you take the paper. Check out that dumb lead editorial on your way downtown."

Jeremy took less than thirty minutes to shower, shave, and dress, then he walked the couple of blocks down Henry Clay to the streetcar stop on St. Charles Avenue. He knew the schedule, and within minutes the boxy green relic came swaying down the tracks, its loud bell clanging as it approached the intersection. The ozone smell of electric sparks sprang from the overhead power source. Jeremy stepped on board and dropped his coins in the coffer. He nodded to the man at the controls, one of the regulars. "Mornin', Roberts."

"Good mornin' to you, Dr. J" the driver said. "a little later than usual, ain't ya?"

"Yeah. We've got a special class today. How're you doing?"

"I'm fine. Jus' fine." Roberts cracked a big smile and shook his head. "What else could a man be on a nice day like this? You have a good un, hear."

"Thanks, Roberts. You, too." Jeremy had always made friends easily, even as a boy. His mother had said his blond good looks and natural charm would catch anybody's eye, but it was more than that. When people discovered his easy-going nature, the disarming way he showed genuine interest in everyone he met, they were hooked.

The streetcar was practically empty and Jeremy took a window seat, leaving room for his notebooks on the hard wooden bench. As the car jostled down the tree-lined boulevard he opened *The Times-Picayune* to the editorial page to read the column that had gotten Dr. Abingdon so fired up:

HEALTH LAW SEGREGATES HIV CARRIERS

With AIDS still running rampant and health professionals unable to stop it, congress finally came to its senses early this year and passed the Health Protection Act of 1989. The HPA becomes the law of the land today, bringing change that is destined to sweep through the social and political fiber of our nation. It mandates a new kind of segregation based upon HIV blood tests, a segregation that is welcomed by this newspaper. though it splits the country right down the middle, this brave new law is the only protection we have against the lethal virus called HIV that is spreading through the population of our land like a wildfire out of control.

Growing fears, fear of death and fear of spiraling health care costs, set the stage for this new tactic, a smart bomb in the war against AIDS.

A slowdown in new cases of AIDS was reported a year or two ago, but that was short lived and, since, then, it has reversed direction as the disease gained a foothold in women, children, and heterosexual men.

Expenditures for health care reached 15 percent of our gross national product in the last fiscal year, yet we still have no cure for AIDS, no way to control the HIV.

The new law requires an annual blood test for HIV, and every citizen must carry an HIV identity card. The card will limit access to designated buildings where transmission of AIDS is considered a high risk. This new kind of segregation will be especially visible in health care facilities.

The federal legislation includes another welcome change, a regional approach to research. Multi-billion dollar funding is provided for three research centers, one of them associated with the Medical Center of Louisiana at New Orleans.

We applaud the Health Protection Act for shielding innocent citizens from the ravages of HIV infection. We agree with the planners who believe a regional focus for research will shorten by years the time it takes to finally identify a safe….

Jeremy's reading was cut short when the streetcar lurched around Lee Circle. He slid toward the aisle and his notebooks hit the floor.

"Sorry, Dr. J," the driver called out. "You gotta watch them curves."

"It's all right, Roberts. I wasn't paying attention." The car jerked through another turn and headed down Carondelet where Jeremy transferred to a bus on the Tulane Avenue route.

The lobby of the medical school was a bustle of activity when Jeremy walked in. The university had set aside the entire day for instructing students about the new monitored entry system and processing their HIV cards. When he spotted a group of his classmates huddled together outside the auditorium, he headed in their direction. "How're you doing, Greg? Mornin', Bob. I guess you won't be staying at Charity, huh?"

Bob shrugged. "Looks that way. I kept hoping the designation would be different, but now we know Charity's positive. What the hell," he said, shrugging, palms up. "Win some, lose some."

That "lose some" comment grated on Jeremy, but he decided to ignore it. "What'll you have to do? How are you supposed to get into another program this late in the year?"

"They told me I'd get an appointment to a negative hospital in a couple of weeks. All I can do is wait and see what the national computer comes up with."

"Too bad," Jeremy said. "I guess a lot of folks'll be in the same boat, one way or the other." All of his classmates knew of Jeremy's needle stick accident and his conversion to HIV-positive.

Bob said, "Yeah, right…same boat. It'll all work out, but it is a royal pain in the ass."

"Really?" Jeremy winked at the others, then turned and grabbed Bob by both his lapels. "Listen to me, buddy. Sounds like you're thinking it's bad news to be HIV-negative. I'd trade with you in a minute."

Bob held up both hands and shook his head. "Whoa—no thanks. No deal there."

"Okay, but you remember that. Make damn sure you remember it when you talk about winning and losing." Jeremy turned away from the group and joined a larger crowd moving into the lecture hall.

For the next two hours the students sat through dull briefings by a series of speakers, most of them with slim claims to expertise on some part of the Health Protection Act. In truth, Jeremy realized, there were no experts—the law was too new.

The last speaker for the day was a physician, a ranking officer of the Public Health Service who first won the group over with a teasing crack about long-winded speakers. Then she said, "Looks like I've got the only good news today. The HPA, as I like to call the new law, has created a network of regional medical centers throughout the country to provide all the health care needs of HIV-positive persons. Your hospital right next door is one of them. Beginning on the first of July all the patients and all the staff of the Medical Center of Louisiana at New Orleans must be blood test positive for the HIV."

She looked around the group before continuing. The students were quiet. "Other hospitals—usually the privately endowed ones—have been identified as HIV-negative facilities. They will not be authorized to treat any patient who is HIV-positive. Every member of their staff must be negative, not only doctors and nurses, but administrators, secretaries, technicians, maintenance workers, housekeepers—everybody."

She shot her eye contact along the front row of students. "The new law also created three regional research institutes and appropriated two billion dollars each to set them up as full-time AIDS research facilities."

She stopped speaking until the low rumble of conversation among the students quieted down. "I'm sure you know one of the three research facilities is to be part of the New Orleans medical complex. All of that hospital's patients will be encouraged to volunteer for testing new drug treatments for HIV. The long wait for FDA approval before human testing of new drugs and new treatments has been waived for all three of the regional institutes—including our own medical center."

She paused, then looked slowly around the room. "New treatment protocols can be tested on volunteer patients as soon as they pass the hospital's local review board. At the discretion of each institute, the second phase of treatment testing may include members of the hospital staff."

That was it. That was exactly what Jeremy wanted to hear. He knew then he had to be at Charity—had to be among the first to receive any up-and-coming HIV treatments. It had to happen soon—all that money and everything. With no good treatment available, not even anything on the drawing board as far as he knew, he had struggled to stay optimistic.

Now, finally, there was hope. Hope made it easier, but not even hope could erase the threat of AIDS, that ugly Sword of Damocles that was always just around the corner, just out of sight. True, some parts of the new law sounded bad, but it held the brightest promise Jeremy'd seen yet and he was determined to make the best of it—determined to take full advantage of being in the right place at the right time.

❖ ❖ ❖

5

Big Charity

SIX WEEKS LATER, ON THE FIRST OF JULY, JEREMY STOOD ON THE Tulane Avenue sidewalk in front of the Medical Center of Louisiana—Charity Hospital. It was the first day of his residency, and he had arrived way too early for the seven AM meeting of new interns. He felt like a little boy, insignificant and nervous about being there as he stared up at the tall, white monolith where he was about to begin five years of surgical training. Early morning was a good time for him, always had been. It was a quiet time, a good thinking time, a time that calmed him.

Looking up at the huge hospital in the soft early light, Jeremy had trouble believing the building was more than fifty years old. Its name had changed a few years earlier, but it was still Big Charity to Jeremy and a lot of other people. Always would be. The hospital's press releases said the governor who built it had a flair for political extremes, but he had dedicated the structure to the medical needs of the people of Louisiana.

The governor's architects and engineers had made sure it represented everything new, twelve shining floors in two side wings topped by another four in the central tower that served as sleeping quarters for the house staff. On dedication day in the thirties, it was a modern new home for an ancient medical institution which had already stood strong through epidemics like yellow fever and typhoid. Jeremy was confident it could do it again—certain it would stand up to today's epidemic as a leading HIV treatment center.

The loud hiss of air brakes dominated background traffic noise and interrupted Jeremy's reverie. He heard approaching footsteps and turned to see Barbara Allison hurrying in his direction from the bus stop at the corner. Barbara was a nurse he'd known for a couple of years. Just known her, that was it, but he'd never forgotten her. She was one of those truly awesome women whose looks had burned into Jeremy's memory the first time he met her. He saw her at parties now and then, but he'd never gotten around to asking her for a date. She was friendly enough, but he had the notion she probably didn't like to go out with medical students, especially not with HIV-positive medical students.

But all that was changed now. He was no longer a medical student, and Barbara was apparently still working at Charity. That meant she must be HIV-positive, too. Maybe it was time to make his move. She was a knockout that morning—smooth suntan under a white uniform, perfect with her light brown hair, her slender figure. And those eyes—big, brown eyes. He thought she worked on one of the medical units…right, cardiology. Probably running late for her shift change report.

Barbara passed without slowing down, but he thought he saw a little smile when she said, "Good morning, Dr. Becker. Welcome aboard."

Unaccustomed to his new title, Jeremy looked around, expecting to see his father. Finally he realized Barbara had spoken to him, and he managed to stammer, "Good morning. Uh...thanks." But it was too late—she had disappeared into the hospital's brand new M-E-P. Everybody knew the controlled entries were called Monitored Entry Points because the lawmakers wanted to avoid words like "controlled" and "regulated." They'd chosen a bright red logo with the letters M-E-P, something easy to recognize.

Jeremy rushed toward the M-E-P, hoping to catch Barbara before she got to the elevator. Unfortunately he had trouble locating his unfamiliar HIV card in the pockets of his equally unfamiliar intern coat. Too much new stuff. He looked at the card, wondering how the tiny magnetic strip could hold so much information. Not only his HIV status, thumb print and standard ID, but also emergency medical data that hospitals could retrieve—blood type, allergies, surgical history, things like that.

Inside the M-E-P booth he inserted the card into a slot that was emphasized by a dim light flashing from inside it. An eye level screen reported:

JEREMY D BECKER
HIV-POSITIVE
EXPIRES: NOV 1994

PLACE YOUR RIGHT THUMB ON
SMALL SCREEN BELOW

Hurrying, Jeremy touched his thumb to the smaller screen. A momentary green flash appeared as the machine read his thumb print.

The door to the hospital lobby did not open as he expected. Instead, a loud, metal-on-metal clanking sound like dead bolts slamming home resonated through the booth. At the same instant an interlocking grid of horizontal steel bars shot out from either side of the opening he'd just entered. Dammit, he was trapped in the stupid booth. Captured. The wailing shriek of an alarm screamed from somewhere outside the booth. A blinding light came on in the ceiling.

What the hell? The briefings hadn't prepared him for this. Sure, they'd talked about capture, but that was supposed to happen to criminals, somebody trying to dupe the system.

An older woman in a nurse aide uniform peered through the bars. "Lordy, doctor, what'd you do to get caught in there like that? Are you all right?"

"I'm okay. I don't know what happened. See if you can get me some help. Get me out of this damn thing."

She slipped an arthritic finger between the bars and pointed to the instruction screen. "Look at that."

The small top window of a split screen flashed in brilliant crimson:

→RED ALERT←

Jeremy leaned closer to read the lower window:

DO NOT PANIC.
YOU WILL NOT BE HARMED.
HELP IS ON THE WAY.

A VIOLATION OF THE HEALTH PROTECTION ACT
HAS CAUSED YOUR CAPTURE.
LAW ENFORCEMENT OFFICIALS WILL ARRIVE
WITHIN 15 MINUTES.

Oh shit. Did they have a surgery residency at Leavenworth?

By that time a crowd had gathered outside the M-E-P and the nurse aide was acting like a hero. He heard her say she had talked to the man inside. "Right up close, face to face. And him a doctor—he oughta know better."

Wait a minute. What about innocent until proved guilty?

Several people pressed around the other door, too, from inside the hospital lobby. He recognized one of them, Lockhart or something, that new administrator who'd been at the briefings. Jeremy couldn't hear them through the door, but the administrator was preening around, waving his arms like he was giving orders to everybody else.

Finally a man in a brown uniform approached from the outside, nudging his big belly right and left to push his way through the crowd. He waved some kind of badge toward Jeremy. "Dugan...U.S. Marshal. Keep your hands where I can see 'em. Stay right where you are."

Then Jeremy saw the gun—a goddamn gun in the man's hand. A gun pointing right at him. What kind of holocaust was this? Lock people in an tiny booth, then come after 'em with guns. Damn thing looked like a cannon when he poked the barrel between the bars.

Dugan stood close to squint inside, his gut pressing against the bars. "What's going on in there? Slip your HIV card out here so I can see it."

"I don't have my card. It's in the machine. Please take that gun away."

Dugan grinned. "Well, well...kept your card did it? Hey, what's that coat you're wearin'? Are you a doctor or somethin'?" He stuffed the pistol into a holster hanging from his gigantic leather belt.

Jeremy pulled an envelope out of his pocket. "I'm supposed to start the surgery residency today. Here's my letter from the hospital. Get me out of here, please—I've got a meeting in thirty minutes."

Dugan fingered Jeremy's letter, then tilted his head back to read through his bifocals. "Dr. Jeremy Becker, huh? Well, doc, let's see what we can do."

He pulled a slender metal rod out of his back pocket. The rod appeared to have a hollow tip, and Dugan used it like a key to open a service door on the outside of the M-E-P booth. "Okay, here's your card. Looks all right to me. Well...what's this? The sensitivity's set way too high on this thing...there, that oughta be better. Stand away from the bars now, I'm gonna open 'er up." The barricades hummed out of sight into the walls of the booth and Jeremy heard the dead bolts move in the inner door.

"Here's your card," Dugan said. "Try it again."

Dubious, Jeremy looked at both sides of the HIV card. "What if it happens again? I'm runnin' out of time."

"It won't do it again—the machine was set wrong. Go ahead."

Jeremy inserted his card then stepped back, expecting the worst. The thumb print message appeared on the screen.

"Put your thumb on there now, and hold it still for a second. That might be what happened before. If you moved your thumb with the sensitivity on max like that, it could've misread the print."

The green light flashed when Jeremy touched the small screen, and the door to the hospital lobby slid open. He grinned. "Thanks, Dugan. Come to see me if you need any surgery."

Dugan put a beefy hand on Jeremy's shoulder. "Get on in there, Doc. That door ain't gonna stay open forever."

Barbara was long gone by the time Jeremy reached the lobby, but at least she didn't see his clown act in the M-E-P. He made up his mind to find a reason to visit the cardiology ward...visit it real soon.

The administrator and his crowd had disappeared, too, so Jeremy stepped around the replica of the state's great seal embedded in the terrazzo floor and took an elevator to the twelfth floor for the interns' orientation meeting. He savored the antiseptic smells that swirled around him as he turned down a long hallway opposite one of the hospital's two Operating Room sections, then headed toward the Delgado Amphitheater at the back of the building.

He walked up a curved flight of stairs to enter the rear of the semicircular amphitheater. Every visible surface in the two-story room was covered with white ceramic tile broken only by pale blue trim tiles. The place put Jeremy in a reverent mood that made him want to keep his voice low in deference to the surgical greats who had held forth there in past teaching demonstrations.

Curved rows of student seats, so steep they seemed to be attached to a vertical wall, were separated from adjacent rows by low, tile-covered barriers. A brightly lighted demonstration area on the lower level included an examining table that appeared so small, so remote, Jeremy felt like he was hovering far above it.

Seeing the amphitheater again brought to mind a recollection that this was where he had learned to do vein punctures. It all started here, he remembered—in medical school, before the hospitals were segregated. This strange looking room had led, in a way, to his own blood test conversion, and now, in an HIV-segregated world, he had come full circle, back to the place where it all started.

6

First Day

Jeremy moved down a side aisle in the Delgado amphitheater on Charity's twelfth floor. He headed toward the lower seats, greeting a few classmates along the way. He spotted Joe Monteleone, a welcome face, the only member of his class he'd known before medical school. Both of them had been competitive swimmers in high school and college, and they had crossed paths from time to time at regional meets. They had first struck up a friendship when Joe said he was from New Orleans, where Jeremy himself had been born during his father's final year at Tulane.

Joe was wiry and dark-haired, the youngest son of proud Italian parents who had immigrated to New Orleans as newlyweds. Over the years Papa Monteleone had established a fine reputation as proprietor of one of the best known Italian delicatessens in the city.

Joe's undergraduate years had been at LSU, on a swimming scholarship, and he had sometimes been matched against Jeremy's University of Texas team. During their early years of medical school at Tulane, Joe and Jeremy had renewed their friendship, occasionally swimming together. More recently, for no particular reason, they had gone separate ways. Jeremy had heard rumors of a Monteleone family conflict—something about Joe having an affair with his father's junior partner. He had considered the rumor nothing more than idle gossip, and he'd chosen to ignore it.

He waved to Joe and moved into the second row to join him. "Morning, Joe. Long time no see. It's great to find a familiar face in this crowd. I didn't know you were taking a residency at Charity." He hesitated. "Come to think of it, I didn't even know you were HIV-positive."

Joe looked embarrassed. "I didn't have any reason to tell you about it, Jeremy. At first I was ashamed of it—didn't want to talk about it at all. Since then I haven't seen much of you."

"Hey, it's okay. Are you still swimming?"

"Not much. Just about gave it up."

"We'll have to take care of that—get you going again. Which residency are you taking?"

"Surgery, same as you."

"Great. We'll probably see a lot of each other." He grinned. "That'll make it easier to get you back in the pool."

Joe looked down at the floor for a long minute before turning back to Jeremy. "Aren't you uncomfortable at the pools? With the HIV and all?"

Jeremy shook his head. "No. The M-E-Ps at the swim clubs are supposed to have negative and positive days, you know."

"I didn't know that. I bet plenty of people still don't like it—afraid of catching AIDS or something."

"Not too many of 'em, Joe. Not anymore. Most of the folks with that mindset have dropped out of the clubs." He grinned. "The rest of 'em know it takes more than chlorinated water to transfer the virus. Let's try to get in some laps next week."

Joe nodded. "I...uh...I heard about your needle stick accident. Rotten luck."

"Yeah, thanks." He wondered whether Joe worried about the things that pestered him like a recurring nightmare. How much time he'd have to practice surgery, whether he'd even finish the residency—worries he'd never mentioned to anybody. Maybe there'd be a time to talk to Joe about that kind of stuff.

Promptly at seven o'clock, a tall, distinguished looking, silver-haired man strode into the amphitheater. He wore a fresh white hospital coat over dark trousers with an Oxford button-down shirt and a blue and gold regimental striped tie.

"Good morning, doctors. My name is Charles Hollander, Director of Medical Education at Charity. By background I am a surgeon." He flashed a sly smile. "But in recent years things changed and I've become a full-time educator. I am especially pleased to welcome all of you to the house staff of a great institution."

Hollander paused and slowly scanned the rows of eager faces filling the amphitheater. "I need to offer the hospital's apologies to one of you. Becker, where are you?"

"Here, sir." Jeremy raised his hand.

Hollander said to the whole group, "Dr. Becker had the dubious honor of being the first person captured by one of our new M-E-P machines. It was a malfunction, Becker. I'm sorry we did that to you on your first day. We'll try not to let it happen again."

"What's he talking about?" Joe asked.

"Later." He could have done without the apology. He'd heard about the hospital grapevine—he'd never keep it quiet now. Barbara would probably figure out he was chasing after her when the damn machine captured him.

As Hollander continued, his candor and his quiet manner quickly identified him to Jeremy as someone he could respect, someone he could go to for advice. "Some of you may be familiar with the VA Hospital, formerly located across the street behind this building. I say 'formerly' because that entire building has now been converted to an HIV Research Institute, part of the Medical Center of Louisiana."

He told them some of the ways their work would involve them in the Institute's AIDS research. That news excited Jeremy—the more involved the better. He was sure everybody in the group felt the same. They all appeared well, but every single one of the new house officers was HIV-positive.

The briefers at the med school had said nobody was certain there'd be enough HIV-positives with the right skills to staff the designated hospitals around the country. But they'd all underestimated the extent of the spreading epidemic. When the mandatory testing started, plenty of people became available, many of them positive on the first test they'd ever had.

Hollander continued. "This will interest you, I'm sure. At this center, we'll be able to avail ourselves of new HIV treatments almost as soon as they come on line." His eyes raced along the residents in the first row. "After short-term toxicity testing in volunteer patients, new treatments will become available to all of you. Any of you may volunteer for Phase II clinical trials, the efficacy trials, without further delay. You'll be able to get any new treatment protocols three to five years sooner than under the old rules."

By late morning the speeches were over and the orientation business was finished. The new residents separated into specialty groups for meetings with their own departments. Socratic teaching began immediately with Surgical Grand Rounds for Jeremy and others in the surgery program. The new residents were the lowest ranking members of the team, and the time at each patient's bedside soon became a grueling quiz with the Chief Resident or attending staff firing questions in rapid succession:

"Who performed the first gastrectomy?"

"In what year?"

"Where did he work?"

"Name three indications for performing gastrectomy."

As if by plan, the Chief resident saved certain questions for the Professor of Surgery—the older residents called him the Chief.

"How does modern treatment for breast cancer differ from Halsted's original operation?"

"At what hospital did Halstead develop his radical mastectomy?"

"Tell us two other contributions Halstead made to modern-day surgery."

Before the questions ended each young resident had learned a new lesson in humility. A defensive unity grew out of the afternoon, the beginning of a camaraderie that would stick with the fledgling surgeons throughout their training years. For this group, the bond was strengthened by knowledge that their very survival might depend upon the success of the AIDS research going on right across the street from their training hospital.

Despite his run-in with the M-E-P system, Jeremy remained confident in the new law. Researchers would find a breakthrough soon, he knew they would. His nagging worries about AIDS seemed less urgent now. He had finally taken the first step toward the only thing he really wanted. On that day he became a surgeon.

7

Operating Room Privileges

Joe Monteleone opened the door quietly. It was a few minutes after five-thirty and early morning light filled the room with a pale glow. Through the windows Joe made out the shapes and flow of New Orleans' streets and downtown buildings stretching fourteen floors below toward the dawn stillness of the Mississippi River waterfront.

He stood motionless for a moment, admiring his sleeping roommate's tousled blond hair, the contour of his slim muscular body covered only by a thin sheet. He smiled at Jeremy's white hospital clothing tossed around the room and knew the guy could only have been asleep for an hour or two. The disarray looked frantic, like a shark's feeding frenzy. That was a sure sign fatigue had driven Jeremy along the quickest path into bed at some time during the night.

The interns' sleeping rooms had been assigned three years earlier, and Joe and Jeremy were listed to share Room 1408. Compatible roommates, they chose to continue the arrangement during their subsequent years of surgery residency. Only rarely did they have in-house duty on the same night, so each of them had the room to himself most of the time.

After the demanding first year of residency they'd decided they needed some place to get away on nights off, a pressure release outside the confining world of the medical center, so they leased a small patio apartment and made it their hideaway. In earlier times the place had been the slave quarters of a fashionable town house. Now it was an efficiency apartment at the rear of one of the old buildings on Burgundy Street in the French Quarter.

Joe had spent the previous night at the apartment and, as often happened, his plans to go out for the evening had been overcome by fatigue. Just as well—he was rested now, ready to tackle another thirty-six hours on duty.

He shook Jeremy gently by the shoulder. His sleepy roommate didn't budge, so he shook harder. "Wake up, Jeremy. Time to get moving."

Jeremy lifted his head. "Morning already? Can't be morning—way too soon." He struggled with a weak smile, then rolled over beneath the sheet. "Thanks, Joe. What a night. Good thing I got an hour or two in the sack before it hit the fan."

"Any good cases?"

"A couple. We started a stomach around midnight—bleeding ulcer, right on top of the gastroduodenal artery. Let me tell you, that sucker can bleed. Then we had a lap that lasted until four-thirty, special delivery from the knife and gun crowd—butcher knife this time. Young guy. Said his friend did it."

Joe laughed. "Seems like it's always a friend. I'd hate to see the ones with enemies."

Jeremy sat up in bed and retrieved his watch from the table, the sheet sliding down his torso as he moved. "Jesus, quarter to six. I better get moving. I'm supposed to meet my new intern for rounds in half an hour." He leaned back against the pillows and beamed. "Then, my friend, I'm going to do my first solo gall bladder. No chief resident, no attending staff. Just my two juniors, assisting me, The Surgeon. Ta, daa...."

"Hey, that's great." Joe rearranged the jumble of clothing and sat in the chair he'd cleared. "I'm ready for something like that myself. I'm just assisting with a couple of hernias this morning. Big deal, huh? I came in early because of my ICU patient—I'm afraid he's getting septic. You remember, that abdomino-perineal Dr. Reynolds did last week."

"You mean, Mr. Gilmore?"

Joe nodded. "You know him?"

"No, but I went by the ICU late last night. Gilmore's a lot better, Joe. Pretty good bowel sounds—his colostomy's starting to work. His fever's down, too. Looks like he's turned the corner. You'll see."

"Thanks for checking on him. I appreciate it." Joe relished the easy going trust between himself and Jeremy. It was the first time he had been entirely comfortable in any kind of one-on-one relationship with another man since his positive HIV blood test.

Jeremy pushed himself out of the bed and walked naked into the bathroom. Joe waited until he heard the toilet flush, then walked in just as Jeremy turned on the water in the shower. Distracted by the hazy view of Jeremy's wet body through the shower door, Joe took a long time brushing his teeth. Finally, shaking the water out of his toothbrush, he peeked over the top of the shower door. "I'm leaving now, Jere. Good luck with your gall bladder."

"Thanks, guy." He flicked water toward Joe's face. "You'll get a good case soon, you'll see."

Joe grinned and turned to leave. "Watch it with the water, wet guy."

"Wait a minute," Jeremy called. "May I borrow a clean white shirt? I'm completely out 'til I pick up my laundry. The one I wore last night is pretty gross."

"Sure, help yourself. There oughta be two or three in my drawer." Joe liked wearing the same size as Jeremy.

The shower door cracked open. "Hey, Joe. One more thing…are you working Friday night?"

Joe stopped and turned back toward the shower. "Yeah, I am. What did you have in mind?"

"Nothing really. I'm going out with Barbara Allison. Thought maybe you'd get a date and join us for dinner." He flashed a wet grin. "On the other hand...as long as you're gonna be in the hospital, I might as well plan on using the apartment after dinner."

Joe laughed. "Sure thing, stud. Plan on it. How long have you been trying to get that beauty in the sack? At least a year, that I know of."

"Longer." Jeremy rubbed a soapy hand over his crotch. "We'll see—she's been pretty friendly lately." He turned back to the steamy spray and closed the shower door. "Get out of here, Joe. I'll see you this evening."

❖

An hour and a half later Jeremy stepped into the operating room where his junior residents were preparing his patient for cholecystectomy, removal of her gall bladder. He moved with an air of authority on this big day, and the circulating nurse spotted him first. "Good morning, Dr. Becker."

Jeremy knew she intended not only to greet him, but to put everybody else in the room on notice that the surgeon was present. Every one of them knew this operation would be his first major case as primary surgeon, with no supervising staff surgeon present. They each deferred to his position as captain of the ship. Jeremy knew exactly what they were doing—he had done it himself many times.

He leaned near his drowsy patient and touched her arm. "Good morning, Mrs. LeCompte. It's Dr. Becker. We're about ready to get started."

The sedated patient struggled to open her eyes. "Dr. Becker. I'm glad to see you. Everybody's been real nice, but I feel better with you here." She managed a half smile before she drifted back into her drugged daze.

Jeremy looked at the eyes of the anesthesiologist, dark brown eyes above his pale blue surgical mask. He raised his own eyebrows in question. Without needing to hear Jeremy's question, the anesthesiologist responded. "Stable on this end. We're all set—want me to put her to sleep?"

Jeremy glanced at the instrument tray, searching for the instruments he preferred among the myriad glistening tools arranged in precise rows on sterile towels. He looked up and found the scrub nurse's quiet gray eyes. "Looks good to me. You ready?"

"Yes, doctor. I have the all instruments you picked."

"Good." He turned back to the anesthesiologist. "Go ahead. I'll scrub."

The intern was already dressed in sterile gown and gloves and he stood near the instrument tray, under the watchful eye of the vastly more experienced scrub nurse. Jeremy signaled the junior resident to join him as he walked into the adjacent scrub room where he methodically scrubbed his hands and forearms with a coarse sterile sponge containing antibacterial soap. He kept an eye on the younger surgeon to be sure that he, too, followed the correct procedure.

The scrubbing ritual was a time honored one, changed little over the years. Aside from its antiseptic purpose, it required time. Time that couldn't be shortened—time that even experienced surgeons often used to organize their thoughts before a planned operation.

But Jeremy didn't need a last minute run-through. He had studied and re-studied every detail of the operation he was about to perform. He had rehearsed a "what-if" algorithm for every unforeseen event he could imagine. He was confident nothing would go wrong, not today. This was the big one for him. He'd waited a long time for it.

Working at his patient's right side, Jeremy directed the team with precision. After a long incision below the patient's right rib cage, he positioned retractors to gently lift her liver and to pull her intestinal tract aside. Then he meticulously removed the woman's gallbladder from the underside of her liver with none of the complications he had rehearsed. A cholangiogram confirmed normal x-ray appearance of the bile ducts, and, some ninety minutes after beginning the operation, he instructed the intern on the fine points of applying a surgical dressing to the wound in the patient's upper abdomen.

Afterward, the junior residents and the anesthesiologist moved Mrs. LeCompte to the post-anesthesia recovery room while Jeremy went to the family waiting area to talk to her husband. He spotted the man sitting alone, gazing out of a window. A cigarette dangled from his yellow-stained fingers. The man looked depressed and frightened, troubled and guilty for some unknown reason. Not at all like the jovial, teasing husband who had tried to reassure his wife the afternoon before.

LeCompte was a small man with rough skin, a ruddy complexion, and dark, unruly hair. Except for a barrel chest, his body appeared shriveled by years of smoking. His sinewy limbs looked oddly powerful—probably the result of hard work on too many shrimp boats in some Cajun town.

Walking toward the window, Jeremy called out, "All finished, Mr. LeCompte. Your wife is fine."

LeCompte rushed toward Jeremy, grasped him by the shoulders and burst into tears.

Jeremy was startled by the man's reaction. He had meant to be reassuring, not frightening. He pulled LeCompte into his arms and held him close.

The distressed man sobbed, "Thank you, doctor! Thank you, God! Thank you, doctor!"

Jeremy said, "It's all right, Mr. LeCompte. She's fine. She'll be ready to go home before you know it. She's in the Recovery Room right now. You can see her when she's back in the ward. Shouldn't be more than two or three hours." He led the man to a chair and guided him into it.

Regaining some composure, LeCompte said, "Dr. Becker, I don't know how I'm ever gonna thank you." He shook his head slowly from side to side. "I did it to her, you know? I already ask God to forgive me, so I ain't worry about that no more. I jus' hope she forgive me. Her and the children." He clutched at Jeremy's hand. "Don't you let that woman die, doctor. I don't know what I would did if somethin' happen to her. I could not stood that."

"Mr. LeCompte, your wife had gallstones. You know that. There is no way you could have caused her gallstones. Where'd you get that idea?"

LeCompte's face twisted in anguish. He rubbed his shoes together and fingered a cigarette out of a pack in his shirt pocket. "I did it, awright. I know I did. My sweet wife was ab-so-lutely fine before I gave her them AIDS. One hundred percent hard working woman. Sweetest thing that ever made a marriage."

"AIDS? Mr. LeCompte, that doesn't—"

"You don't have to say nothin'. I know I did it. I don't know exactly when I got the AIDS myself, but I sure gave 'em to her. You see, a few years ago, while she was carryin' our baby girl, I got drunk a few times an' ended up in a whorehouse." He lighted the cigarette he'd been playing with. "God's punishin' me. Hell, I had the AIDS the first time they tested us for 'em." New rivers of tears ran down his face. "So did she, doctor. So did she. That por sweet woman."

Finally Jeremy understood. He lowered his voice. "Listen, LeCompte, your wife might have gotten the AIDS virus from you, the HIV. She probably did. But she does not have AIDS. Neither do you." He gripped LeCompte's arm. "That virus has nothing to do with her gallstones—nothing at all. With any luck we'll have a cure for the virus before either one of you develops AIDS—a long time before."

A Red Cross worker looked into the room, and Jeremy motioned her over to sit with LeCompte. "I'm going to leave now, Mr. LeCompte. I need to get back to the Recovery Room. I'll look for you downstairs on the ward when I make rounds this evening."

Sobbing quietly, the unhappy man waved in Jeremy's general direction.

In the Recovery Room, the Charge Nurse told Jeremy Mrs. LeCompte was stable and starting to react from her anesthesia. He spotted the junior resident at the desk, probably writing orders in the patient's chart, and the intern held up a vial of blood he had drawn for post-operative lab studies.

The hospital's perennial shortage of lab technologists still delegated blood drawing to interns or medical students. Jeremy remembered his own earlier years—that kind of scut work was the worst. He tried not to think too much about all the trouble blood drawing had caused him as a medical student.

"Thanks for your help, guys," he said as he joined the others. "You were great."

The junior resident beamed. "We ought to thank you, Jeremy. That operation was slick as a spritz of WD-40."

Jeremy grinned. "Yeah, it was nice—thanks to you two." He paused. "Listen, I need to tell you about something odd that just happened. Mrs. LeCompte's husband believes he caused her gallstones by giving her HIV and it's got him pretty upset. Talk to him about it when you see him on the ward."

The junior resident frowned. "Weird. Where do people get crazy ideas like that. We'll try to set him straight."

"Don't be surprised if you can't change his mind—he's a hard-headed Cajun. Just take it easy with him. Help him work it out." Jeremy looked at the wall clock. "You two better get back to the OR. The Chief must be about ready to start the thyroid. Get going—I'll look after Mrs. LeCompte. Remember Rule One, we don't keep the Chief waiting—not ever."

They both laughed and turned to leave. "Got it. See you in the clinic this afternoon, okay?"

Jeremy examined Mrs. LeCompte to satisfy himself she was stable. Reassured, he caught up with the nurse at another patient's bedside. "Thanks for your help with Mrs. LeCompte, Hillary. I'm going up to Room 1408 to rest for a while. Please call me for any change in her condition—anything at all."

Still riding the high of his big case, he bounded up the two flights of stairs to the fourteenth floor and got the room door half open before he heard his roommate's voice. "Dammit, still busy. Everybody in Orleans Parish must be calling Dr. Reynolds. Friggin' private practice...."

Joe hung up the phone just as Jeremy opened the door. "Jeremy. I didn't expect you at this time of day. I'm glad you're here—I've got big trouble. Mr. Gilmore died this morning."

"Gilmore? Your patient in the ICU?"

"Right. He was doing better, like you said. Then his fever spiked around seven o'clock, just about the time I got there. In half an hour his blood pressure was down. An hour later he was dead. I was right there the whole time. I did everything, but I couldn't stop it. Nothing made a bit of difference."

"Damn. What do you think happened?"

"That's the problem…I don't know. The nurses told me he was stable for the rest of the night after you saw him. They thought he was finally getting a solid night's sleep, so when the lab tech came to draw his blood culture at four AM they sent him away. They wouldn't let him wake Mr. Gilmore—told the tech to come back later. He did come back, and he drew the blood culture around six o'clock."

"Blood culture? Joe, I cancelled that order for blood cultures. Gilmore looked so good last night, I didn't think he needed any more. Who ordered another one—especially at four AM? I thought you said his fever spiked at seven."

"I don't know who ordered it. Your team was in house—must have been one of them."

"I don't think so. All of us were in the OR most of the night."

"Maybe the clerk sent the lab slip in early—before you cancelled the order."

"Come on, Joe. I cancelled that order in plenty of time. I told the nurse about it, too." He shook his head. "Man, I'm gonna chew that woman out. She should have—"

"Don't do anything, Jeremy. It's my patient, I'll ask the nurses about it. The culture may help us anyway. It was drawn about an hour before Gilmore started to go downhill. They're gonna do an autopsy, but that blood culture may our best clue to what happened."

Jeremy realized it was time to back off, let Joe run his own show. "I'm damn sorry he died, Joe. He looked so much better...."

Joe's face twisted into a pained grimace. "Shit, I don't even know why Gilmore died. It was hard enough explaining that to his wife. Now I've got to tell Dr. Reynolds about it, and you know how picky Reynolds is."

"Really." Jeremy put his hand on Joe's shoulder. "You do know there was nothing else you could have done, don't you? You must know that."

Joe nodded.

"Then don't let Reynolds get to you. Just convince him you covered all the bases—he'll be all right."

Joe doodled a matrix of bold Xs on the note pad beside the telephone. "Easy to say. I'm the one who's got to talk to Reynolds. You know he'll give me grief over it."

"Listen," Jeremy said, "let me present my findings from last night at the next death conference. I could tell the staff how much better Gilmore was a few hours before he went bad. I was there, Joe. I saw it."

Joe shook his head. "Thanks, Jeremy. You don't need to do that. I can handle it." Suddenly he grinned. "Hey, I almost forgot. How'd your gall bladder go this morning?"

A proud smile lighted Jeremy's face. "Great case—could not have been better. Not a single problem, right out of the textbook. I just left her in the Recovery Room. Stable as a rock."

8

Dark Corridors

THE AFTERNOON CLINIC WAS BUSY, NEARLY TWICE THE USUAL number of patients. Unexpectedly late when he and the team finally saw the last patient, Jeremy hurried to his room to pick up his dirty clothes. Putting off his own laundry until the day's work was completely finished was exactly the reason he was already borrowing clean shirts from Joe. That was a problem he intended to change. He thought he could still make it before the hospital laundry closed—with a little luck, and if the elevators weren't too busy,

Arms loaded with his soiled white pants and shirts, he rushed along the back corridors of the huge building's basement. Hurrying past the tunnel that had once been a popular pedestrian link between the hospital and the next door medical school, he sensed something was wrong. Something was out of place. The tunnel door—what the hell? Not a soul in sight, but the door was open.

That made no sense at all. They'd sealed off the tunnel when the Health Protection Act became law and Charity Hospital was designated an HIV positive facility. The monitored entry system had stopped that access to the building. They'd blocked each end of the tunnel with a heavy steel wall, leaving only a locked fire door in each end of the tunnel for emergency use. That's what grabbed Jeremy's attention—not only was the emergency door at the tunnel entrance unlocked, but for some reason the door was half open.

That corner of the hospital basement was dark and little used. The corridor near the old tunnel had always seemed threatening to Jeremy, but this time it seemed especially dank and clammy. The blocked tunnel reminded Jeremy of the "big brother" elements of the Health Protection

Act, and the open tunnel door heightened the sinister mood of the place. Jeremy thought about stopping to check it out, but he'd miss the laundry if he did. Later, he decided—he'd check it out later. After the laundry. He was practically there anyway.

A young woman with tightly curled dark hair was at work behind the counter in the laundry's small anteroom. A little overweight, she was chewing gum, and she wore way too much makeup. Jeremy thought she was probably trying to hide the fading traces of acne still visible on her cheeks. She ignored his arrival, just kept on adding up the day's accounts, or whatever she was doing. Probably getting ready to close for the day.

He waited, until finally the craziness of it became more than he could tolerate…rushing down here, spotting what looked like a violation of hospital security, then being forced by the minimum-wage employee to stand around cooling his heels. "Pardon me," he said. "Do you have a key to those tunnel doors out there?"

Annoyed, the woman glared up from her ledger, then saw who it was and softened a little. The rapid-fire rhythm of her gum chewing slowed down to a normal pace. "Yeah, we've got a key. We've got the only key. Opens both ends. I keep it in the cash drawer, but you'll have to get a letter from the front office if you wanna use it."

"I don't need the key. I just want to let you know something weird—"

Like many low level functionaries, the woman ran for cover when she sensed blame coming her way. "We don't even use the darn key unless there's a fire or somethin'. That old tunnel's in our emergency plan. Look for yourself, the plan is right over there on the bulletin—"

The rest of her words were lost in a loud hiss of steam that rushed with a starchy smell from the workroom behind her.

Jeremy decided he understood well enough, and he didn't like the frame of mind he'd gotten into. He was thinking like Sam Abingdon or somebody…like his own father. The laundry attendant was just an unfortunate woman with too little education and too little opportunity. She must have unlocked the emergency door for some reason—that's all there was to it. Already late for his team's evening rounds, he signed for his clean clothes and got out of the hot, noisy place as quickly as he could.

But when he passed the tunnel entry again he stopped dead in his tracks, flabbergasted by what he saw. The fire door was closed. This time he tested the door, and the damn thing was locked. Wait a minute. He'd been in the laundry—nobody came in there, nobody returned the key. The laundry woman said she had the only key. How in the hell...?

He heard footsteps and looked up to see the outline of a dark-haired man shuffling down the corridor. Looked like he was wearing gray coveralls, the hospital's utility uniform for housekeeping and maintenance workers. Something familiar about him, but Jeremy couldn't quite figure out who he was. He remembered seeing that same guy around the patient wards with a housekeeping cart. Leonard something. What was it? Cajun name....Guidry, that was it. Leonard Guidry. Probably going off duty at that time of day.

Walking faster, Jeremy called, "Guidry, wait up a minute. Did you see anybody coming out of the old tunnel?"

"No." Guidry said.

He sounded a little too quick, a little too emphatic to suit Jeremy.

Guidry paused half-way through the door to the men's locker room. He cracked a big smile and said, "Ain't nobody down here, doc, but you and me. I'm goin' off duty, and I don't reckon you been in the tunnel. That door been locked for two, three year, anyway."

What the hell, Jeremy decided, no harm had been done. Still, something was not right. Guidry didn't act concerned about the security breach. Well, the emergency door was locked again, and there was no sign of damage in the area. "Okay, Guidry. Have a good night." He pushed the whole business out of his mind and took an elevator to the fourth floor to catch up with his team.

Evening rounds were more complete, more formal, than their early morning walk-through. Jeremy hung his clean laundry in the nurses' station, then he, the junior residents and medical students stopped at every patient's bed, not just the ones who had problems. This was the day the chief resident made rounds with the team, and the head nurse joined them, too. Jeremy sometimes wondered if the patients were scared stiff by the imposing group in white coats parading through the wards.

The interns usually presented each patient, one of the group examined the appropriate body part, then, still at the bedside, they reviewed the day's laboratory results and x-ray films. The medical students and interns fielded the group's questions about each patient's condition, and together they fine-tuned each treatment plan. Jeremy had never liked all that talk right at the bedside. The patients couldn't understand half of it and they were usually ignored, like they weren't even there. Whenever they came to his own patients, he worked at keeping them involved—after all it was their well-being the team discussed.

When the group stopped beside the patient whose gall bladder Jeremy had removed earlier in the day he interrupted the routine. Touching the woman's arm, he said, "Mrs. LeCompte is a special patient.

I'll present her." He reviewed her history, then described the operation he had performed. The junior resident examined her abdomen, the group checked the lab studies, and concluded she was heading for an uncomplicated recovery. Richard MacLeod, the chief resident drew Jeremy aside and congratulated him. "She really looks great, Jere. Hard to tell she had a major operation a few hours ago."

Words like that from the chief resident were the best ego boost Jeremy could hope for. On the way to the next ward, he detoured into a side hallway. "I need to stop by waiting room. I'll catch up with you on 4-B."

The corridor leading to the family waiting room was dark at that time of day, but the man he was looking for, his patient's husband, was easy to spot in the room itself. Once again he was sitting alone, near the window, surrounded this time by a dense cloud of cigarette smoke.

"Mr. LeCompte," Jeremy said, holding out his hand. "How're you doing tonight? We just saw your wife—she's doing great."

LeCompte shook Jeremy's hand. "Thank you, Doctor. The nurse told me she was okay, but I don't know...she look so pale to me."

"That's normal," Jeremy said, but LeCompte still looked skeptical. "Trust me, it's temporary. Just an after-effect of the anesthesia and everything. She'll look a lot better in the morning. You'll see."

"Well...okay, doctor." Hesitating, LeCompte pulled a cigarette from his shirt pocket and fumbled with a time-worn Zippo lighter. "Doctor Becker, I am real sorry for the way I act this mornin'."

"Don't worry about it. You were concerned about your wife, that's all. Nothing wrong with that. You just let your emotions run away from you."

"I sure did that. Comes from bein' a full-bleed Cajun, I guess." A weak smile ran across LeCompte's face, then faded. "Hearin' what you say makes me feel better, but I guar-an-tee I am ashamed for givin' her them AIDS." He shook his head and flattened his cigarette in an overflowing ashtray. "I wish I could take the pain for her, Doctor. Like I'm told you, she's a good woman. I'd do anything to relieve her sufferin'."

Jeremy gripped the man's shoulders. "That's nice, LeCompte—a good way to feel about your wife. Just don't forget what I told you this morning about AIDS." He looked into the man's exhausted eyes. "Listen, why don't you go on home now? Get some rest. She'll be fine tonight. You can see her early in the morning."

"I'll be leavin' soon. Her sister's comin' to sit up with her."

Jeremy knew there'd be no way to dissuade the woman's family from having at least one relative in the hospital day and night while she was there, but he tried. "Her sister doesn't need to do that—no one needs to be here. We'll take good care of her for you."

The man shook his head. "I know y'all will, but the women want to be here…just in case she needs somethin', ya know." He peered into a half-empty coffee cup, then pulled out another cigarette instead. "It's awright, doctor. Her sister's got a pos'tive blood test. She can get in here without no trouble."

Jeremy had learned that the HIV entry restrictions made "sitting up" in hospitals difficult for some families. As a result, enterprising support groups, both HIV-positive and HIV-negative groups, had sprung up. They were like surrogate families who, for a fee, would represent loved ones of different HIV status. Volunteer support groups were available, but he'd noticed many families preferred to pay for the service, a bizarre exorcism of guilt like some cultures that hired professional mourners for a funeral.

❖❖❖

9

New Hope, New Suspicions

THE TEAM HAD FINISHED WITH THE PATIENTS BY THE TIME Jeremy reached the next ward. He found them in the conference room, Rich MacLeod talking from a podium at the front of the room. Jeremy slipped into a seat just in time to hear MacLeod say, "The Chief asked me to pass along some good news. The latest experimental treatment coming out of the HIV research group looks promising. Very promising."

A collective groan rose from the group. "Oh, no, not again. We hear that every time."

MacLeod grinned and continued. "No, I mean it. This one looks better than anything they've come up with yet. It's a gene splicing technique that could stop the virus in its tracks. The researchers say their *in-vitro* results were a lot better than they expected. They tested the treatment against a hyper-virulent HIV strain they've isolated, but that's another story—it's a strain that's more lethal than anything ever recovered from a living patient."

First I've heard of that, Jeremy thought. A new strain? Some kind of super-virus? Everybody else in the group looked puzzled, so he concluded it was new to them, too.

"The new treatment dramatically slows down the rate of virus mutation," MacLeod said. "May even stop it completely—stop the genetic changes that allow HIV to develop drug resistance." He drew an elongated cell on the blackboard, then highlighted its surrounding membrane with yellow chalk. "It works by inhibiting an enzyme in the virus cell membrane. It looks good in the lab, but it's never been tested in human subjects. The usual double-barreled, two-stage test protocol is the next step—see if it's safe, then see if it works." He held up his hand, "First they'll stop virus mutation,..." and guided the chalk into it like a missile, "then give their new drug to kill the virus."

MacLeod stopped and looked around the group. "Pretty nice, huh? They've just put the final touches on the clinical protocol, and that's where we come in—the Chief wants us to really push our patients to volunteer for testing this one. If it's as good as they hope, the two-stage treatment could be available for us in less than a year."

"Why can't we get it now?" a medical student asked. "I'll volunteer."

"We have to look at toxicity first, MacLeod explained. "The initial phase of clinical trials always looks at human toxicity. Before we can take the treatment ourselves, before the efficacy trials begin, we have to enroll enough volunteers to complete the toxicity testing. Toxicity testing is Phase I, but that won't take long—not with you guys signing up the patients."

Boisterous comments erupted around the room:

"All right!"

"Go for it."

"Great news. About time, too."

"Hey, maybe we will get to practice surgery before we die of AIDS."

When the commotion died down MacLeod dismissed the team and asked Jeremy to go to the ICU with him for a final look at the team's most critical patients. "Let the juniors go ahead. It'll take 'em a couple of hours to get the patients ready for tomorrow's surgery. We can work faster in the ICU without them, anyway." He grinned. "I don't know about you, but I'm ready to get out of here."

Jeremy was all for that. His duty day had begun more than thirty-six hours earlier. But fatigue did not dull his enthusiasm for the new treatment protocol. He wanted to hear more. "What else did the Chief say, Rich? About that new treatment for HIV? Sounds like he's pretty excited about it."

MacLeod nodded. "He is excited." He scratched the stubble of dark red beard on his chin and led Jeremy into the elevator. "I am, too. It's time for me to make some decisions about going into practice next year. I'd sure like to do it without worrying about AIDS cutting me off at the pass."

"Yeah, I know what you mean," Jeremy said. "Every new treatment we've seen for the past couple of years has turned out to be nothing more than temporary improvement. Seeing that happen again and again depresses the hell out of me. Sometimes I have to hide my frustration from the junior residents—if those guys stop preaching volunteer testing to our patients, we may never solve the damn puzzle."

"You're right there, Jeremy, but this one really does look good. You realize it's a whole new approach? None of the other centers is on this track yet. Inhibiting virus mutation to slow down drug resistance just may be the break-through we've been waiting for. The research group is giving it a full court press. Some of 'em are even talking about a Nobel prize."

Jeremy raised his eyebrows. "Impressive. From what you said, it sounds like that new super-virus has a lot to do with it. What are they calling the new strain, anyway? If our guys discovered it, don't they get to name it?"

"Yeah, they do. The genetic engineers actually invented it with some of their fancy techniques. There's only one thing about it that's different from the standard AIDS virus. It multiplies and it mutates almost a thousand times faster than any naturally occurring HIV strain."

"A thousand times faster? That means testing each new protocol can be completed a hell of a lot quicker, doesn't it? Something like time compression?"

"That's it. That's the whole secret. They're gonna call their super-bug HIV, NOLA strain."

"NOLA strain?"

"Yeah, like that old song—New Orleans L-A.

Jeremy smiled. "I bet their cultures of the NOLA strain are guarded like Fort Knox. Can you imagine how fast AIDS would move in a patient infected with that aggressive strain?"

"Really. You oughta go over there, Jeremy. See their new techniques for yourself. I think you'd be impressed—I know you'd be enthusiastic about the new clinical trials."

"Hey, I'd like to. Ask the Chief to get me a clearance, will you?" Jeremy pulled out his pocket calendar. "How about next Thursday afternoon?"

"No problem," MacLeod said. "I'll ask the Chief tomorrow. He can set it up with one phone call."

When they reached the ICU nurses' station, Jeremy was surprised to see Leonard Guidry, that housekeeper from the basement. He was looking intently at the bright red clip board which listed the names and diagnoses of all the patients in the unit. The man's cleaning cart was nearby—it could be innocent. Still...Guidry had said he was going off duty.

"Hey, Guidry," Jeremy said. "What're you doing? Looking for a friend on the patient list?"

The housekeeper looked guilty as sin, just like he did in the basement, like he wanted to disappear or something. Jeremy remembered a long-ago morning when his own father walked into his room without knocking. Caught him masturbating. He remembered feeling guilty, burning hot guilty, yet trying to act like nothing had happened. That was the way Guidry was acting.

Guidry glanced up with a dumb-looking smile and held out the clip board toward Jeremy. "Naw, the board jus' fell down when I picked up the trash can. I can't figure out which hook to put it on."

"Just put it on the desk," MacLeod said. "Anywhere there is okay. Dr. Becker and I need to do our work here."

MacLeod's tone made his impatience very clear. Guidry gathered up his cleaning paraphernalia, in a hurry now to get out of the way.

Jeremy pulled the housekeeper aside to question him privately while MacLeod looked through a patient's chart. "What are you doing up here, Guidry. I thought you were going off duty when I saw you in the basement. That's what you told me."

Guidry glanced around the room. "I was leavin', Dr. Becker, but...uh...one of the night men called in sick, and...and I took his shift." He began to talk faster. "I can sure use the extra pay. I sorta like the night shift anyway. Everything's quiet, ya know? At night, you'll got to be your own boss most of the time."

Guidry's life seemed so simple—his explanation so reasonable. Watching the man push his cart slowly into the hallway and leave the ICU, Jeremy wondered why hospital support workers always had something to push. For them it was a hallmark, like the doctors' white coats. Didn't seem to matter what they pushed…a cart or a bucket, a small table or a bed. Anything would do. Anything that made them look official like they were on a mission of some kind. Maybe Guidry was on some personal mission—hard to tell, sometimes, about those Cajun guys.

❖ ❖ ❖

10

Jeremy Remembers

As the night wore on Dr. Becker refined his handwritten yellow pad notes to a computer document which would later become the draft of his keynote address at the AIDS conference. The work caused him to fall into a melancholy mood of remembering, reminiscing, thinking about some of the good things and some of the bad things that had become part of his everyday life during the years of the Health Protection Act.

Jeremy's drifting thoughts brought to mind his excitement about visiting the HIV research facility and the prospect of seeing firsthand the early stages of an evolving treatment protocol which had held the best hope to that time of getting the damn HIV out of his own body.

For some reason his wandering mind recalled that housekeeping worker at Charity, Guidry, that was his name, the guy he'd run across in the dark basement corridor near that old tunnel. The same guy who'd showed up unexpectedly in the ICU when Jeremy and the chief resident were making rounds.

Guidry was a recurring figure in many of the things that came down the pike during those years when everybody at Charity was distracted by the spreading wildfire of AIDS that was sweeping across the country. Jeremy wondered what kind of early life Guidry had—what could have produced a man who seemed unable to distinguish right from wrong. He'd learned Guidry grew up in the small southern Louisiana town of Thibodeaux—down in the bayou country south of New Orleans. That guy must have had quite a boyhood to become the man Jeremy had tangled with.

His thoughts were interrupted by a faint knock at the door of his study. He turned to see Barbara come in wearing a lightweight blue housecoat over white silk pajamas. She smiled a greeting, then padded barefoot to his desk and put her hands on his shoulders. "How's it going, Jere? I finished my book, but I couldn't fall asleep knowing you were in here working your fingers to the bone. I don't know any way I can help you with it, but if there's anything I can do…. Oh heck, what I really mean is, can't you finish that darn speech later?"

Jeremy said, "I need to keep going, Barb. I'm on a roll right now and I might lose it if I quit working."

She glanced over his shoulder at the computer screen. "Looks like a pretty good start to me." She read the last paragraph he had written. "Hmm, that's real good. What's next? Where are you going with it from here?"

"I haven't decided yet. I was thinking about some of the things that happened to us at Charity, and I happened to remember that housekeeper, that Cajun housekeeper named Guidry."

"That bastard! Surely he's not going to be part of your speech. He's the one who caused a lot of the troubles we had in those bad years. Can't we just forget about Guidry and everything he did?"

11

Lennie

THE BOY STOOD BACK FROM THE FRONT WINDOW, JUST BEHIND one of the limp curtains that hung at each side. His mama sent him there whenever she saw a stranger coming. His lookout post, she called it, where he could see the whole front yard and hear everything that happened. He was s'posed to run out through the back door and get help if there was any kind of trouble.

Mama had seen the big Lincoln pull up on the road in front of the house—that's why she'd sent Lennie to his lookout. She stood just inside the front door, safe behind the latched screen, waitin' for whoever was in that big car to come up on the porch. She propped the shotgun in the corner by the door, out of sight from the porch but close enough to reach if she needed it.

The boy and his mother had been here alone in the weeks since his daddy died. A lot of strangers came at first. Insurance men, bill collectors and such. They didn't come much anymore, but his mama kept their lookout plan goin'. He had to come straight home from school every day to help her with it. She told him she was scared of strangers—needed a big boy like him to look after her.

Shoot, she'd been scared as long as he could remember. She was scared to death of Daddy, not that he could blame her for that, the way he hit her all the time. But that wouldn't happen anymore.

He remembered seeing that same black Lincoln in town now and then, but he didn't know the man who got out of it. He looked important, though, coming up the steps. Him wearin' a felt hat, fancy suit, and all that.

From behind the screen door Mama said, "Evenin', Mr.

Boudreaux."

The man took off his hat. "Miz Guidry."

"Can I help you?"

"I came to see your boy. I'd like to talk to him a while, if he's here."

"Why would a man like you want to talk to an eleven year old boy? It ain't more trouble is it?"

He saw the man shake his head.

"Did the sheriff send you? He already talked to the boy, you know. Three times he talked to him. Had the po' boy so strung out he couldn't even sleep."

"It's not any kind of trouble, Miz Guidry. I want to talk to the boy about doin' some chores at Rena's house."

"Your sister, Rena?"

"Yes, ma'am. He could stop by Rena's for a little while after school every day, then come in on Saturday mornin'. I'd pay him for the work. It's the least I can do—losing his daddy and all."

Mama wiped her mouth with the back of her hand. She unlatched the screen door and pushed it open to step out on the porch. "What kinda work? I'd want him home before dark."

"Nothing hard. Cut the grass, rake up leaves in the fall, bring in wood for the fireplace, things like that. Maybe run to the drugstore now and then for Rena."

"What about that darkie that lives with her?"

"You mean Lucifer?"

"Yeah. Why can't he do for your sister?"

"Lucifer's too old to do much, Miz Guidry. He's been with Rena forty years—that's the only reason I keep him on. She's the nearest thing he's got to a family. He still drives her car when she wants to go somewhere. Looks after that old car real good, too, and makes sure the house runs like it ought to. But his knees are bad and he can't do the outside work anymore. That's why I want to hire your boy. Can I talk to him?"

"Why can't you jus' talk to me 'bout it? How much do you want to pay him?"

"Let me talk to the boy—man to man, you know. That'd be best for him. With his daddy gone, he needs to start lookin' after things for himself. I hear he's right smart for his age."

"You been checking up on him?"

"I talked to the school principal. He told me Lennie gets along pretty good in school."

Still standing at the window, the boy could see that softened Mama up a little. She sat down in her rocking chair and waved toward the swing for the man to sit down.

"His grades are good enough, I guess" Mama said, "but he has to work at it. Lennie seems to like school a lot. Lord knows where he got that. Not from his daddy I guarantee."

The man leaned forward, holding his hat by the brim with two hands. "Miz Guidry, I understand your husband was a mean man."

Mama stopped rocking. "He was a hard man, not really mean. Always wanted more than he could find a way to get. He took it out on me and the boy sometimes."

"Didn't you have another son? What ever became of him?"

"I did have another boy, two years older than Lennie. He died in 1967, the same year Lennie was born."

The man shook his head. "Shame. Two years old. Was he sickly?"

"Never had been. You know, it's a mystery to me why that young'un died. I was right here in Thibodaux when it happened." She looked away and dabbed at her eyes with a handkerchief. "I was in the hospital after givin' birth to Lennie."

The man nodded. "Damn shame."

"I was so sick I didn't know anything for two, three weeks." Mama glanced toward the front window, then held her hand to the side of her mouth and tried to whisper. "I'd had a hard birth. The midwife couldn't take care of it, that's why I was in the hospital. When I came home the older boy was dead. Some kinda accident, my husband said."

"Is that all he told you?"

"Just about. We had a mule at that time. He said the mule rolled over on the boy. Got real mad every time I asked him about it, so I jus' kept quiet. It wouldn't help the boy none, I figured. He was gone. My husband shot the mule."

"You never had another baby?"

She shook her head. "The doctor said another one'd kill me. They tied my tubes after Lennie's birth."

"Well, we just have to make Lennie into a boy you can be real proud of." He pulled a gold watch out of his pocket and looked at it, then wound the stem a couple of times. "You gonna let me talk to him?"

"You can talk to him, Mr. Boudreaux. Just be easy with him, he's a good boy. His daddy never did treat him right." She stood up and took a few steps toward the front window. "Come on out here, Lennie. Mr. Boudreaux wants to talk to you."

Boudreaux grinned. "He heard the whole thing, didn't he?"

Mama nodded her head.

"Why don't you leave us alone when he comes out here. I won't let him agree to anything until he talks to you about it."

"Awright, Mr. Boudreaux. I'll be in the kitchen." She turned and opened the screen door for Lennie to come out before she went inside.

"Come over here, Lennie," Boudreaux said. "Come sit on the swing with me."

The boy didn't feel right around grown men—especially strangers. "That's awright. I'll jus' sit over here in my mama's chair."

Boudreaux looked him over from head to toe. "You're a big boy for eleven, Leonard Guidry. Is that right, you're eleven years old?"

"Yessir. Born in 1967."

"You heard what your mama and me were talking about?"

"Yessir."

"I want you to work for me, Lennie. You heard me talking about that, didn't you?"

The boy nodded. "Where do you live?"

Boudreaux leaned back and moved the swing a little bit. "Well, I live in New Orle'ns. I want you to work at my sister's house right here in Thibodaux, but you'd be working for me. Understand?"

"Yessir. Miss Rena's your sister?"

"That's right. Miss Rena Boudreaux. Lives in that big house at the end of Oak Street. You know her, don't you?"

"I seen her ridin' down the street in that old car the colored man drives." He knew her all right. The older boys, Raymond and those, had told him the big old shiny car was a Packard. It was so quiet you couldn't tell it was runnin', like she was sneaking up on you or something. They called her the stone lady. Said she couldn't move around too much by herself. The colored man had to pick her up to put her in or out of the Packard.

"Lennie, the colored man is called Lucifer. He works for Miss Rena, too, but I need you to do some different jobs. Jobs he can't do any more. I know I can count on you to take care of things for me."

Lennie didn't know what to say. The idea of being right in the house with the stone lady was creepy, but he knew Mama needed the money.

"I come down here to Thibodaux every week, Lennie. On Thursdays. I'd pay you twenty-five dollars a week if you take the job."

Lord, that was more money than he'd ever dreamed of having at one time. "When would you want me to start?"

Boudreaux looked at his gold watch again. "We could go over there right now. Just to show you around the place, tell you what I want you to do and all. You can start working tomorrow after school if you want to."

Twenty-five dollars a week—he'd be rich. "I don't know, Mr. Boudreaux...I'll have to ask my mama."

"Go ask her now. Tell her I'll get you back before supper."

Lennie jumped up and ran toward the front door.

"Wait a minute, Lennie. There's something else."

"Yessir?"

"My first name is Marshall. That's what I want you to call me."

The idea of calling a grown man by his first name made him uneasy until he thought of a way out of it. Then he beamed. "Okay, Mr. Marshall. I'll be right back."

12

A Night Off

TWO DAYS LATER, ON FRIDAY, JEREMY ARRANGED FOR Rich MacLeod to cover for him during the team's evening rounds. He wanted plenty of time to get ready—wanted no reason to hurry, no rush about getting ready for his dinner date. Surgery residents were always exhausted, and he remembered an embarrassing time when he'd fallen asleep during dinner at a quiet restaurant. He did not want that to happen again. The plans for this night off were much more ambitious than falling asleep—Barbara deserved a lot more than that. Maybe he'd make time for a quick nap before going out.

When he left the hospital the worst of the afternoon heat had passed, and the French Quarter unveiled its unique air of mystery that Jeremy enjoyed. He didn't always get that special feeling from the Quarter, but when he did it was a good omen, like all the ghosts of the *Vieux Carre* were watching over him. Tonight was no exception. Within minutes he had the good luck to find a parking space on Burgundy Street less than a block from the apartment.

The heavy wrought iron gate at the sidewalk entrance to the old red brick building looked more like it might lead to a cell rather than to the refuge it represented to Jeremy and his roommate. Jeremy unlocked the gate and walked into a dark, narrow passageway cooled by evaporating moisture from the ancient bricks. The main house rose three stories on the left and, on the right, thick vines covered a high brick wall. Damp, moldy bricks underfoot completed the tunnel-like passage which was completely enclosed except for a tiny patch of sky far above, too tiny to admit more than a few minutes of sun each day. Street noises were muffled by the tight passage. A bright opening at the far end pulled

Jeremy away from the musty air of the entry. The welcoming sounds of a splashing fountain urged him toward the open space beyond.

The courtyard was a forest of tall potted plants that gave privacy to each of the building's three apartments. Large plants thrived in the sultry heat and gave the place a natural, tropical appearance, and fresh garden smells dominated. Red hibiscus bloomed next to the wall on the sunny side of the patio, and flame-colored bougainvillea struggled to climb the bricks of the main house. A clump of banana trees sprawled at the back, near the door to the old slave quarters. Tubs and pots of brilliant-leaved crotons, rubber plants, and birds-of-paradise were everywhere, and baskets of spidery ferns hung above them. In the center of it all the gentle sounds of the fountain created an island in the sea of rich foliage, an island that invited relaxed conversation.

Jeremy barely knew his nearest neighbors, the young couple who lived on the ground floor of the main house. They worked nights at the Royal Orleans Hotel, and spent most days as street vendors of the paintings and book bindings they created. Their friends were the artists and artisans who always set up shop around Jackson Square or in Pirate's Alley next to St. Louis Cathedral.

The nominal caretaker of the place was Henry Valadon, a young attorney whose spacious flat filled the upper two floors of the main house. Jeremy had discovered Henry's wrought iron balcony overlooking Burgundy Street was a great spot for viewing the neighborhood architecture, or for watching the insane crowds in the street below during Mardi Gras.

Henry was sitting alone beside the fountain when Jeremy arrived. He looked half-asleep, probably hypnotized by the late afternoon heat and the steady gurgling of the fountain. "Oh, hi, Jeremy," he said. "You're early today." He stirred the ice in a large ceramic pitcher. "How about a glass of sangria?"

"Looks like you could use some help with it all right. That's a lot of sangria for one person."

Henry laughed, then stood up and stretched. "The friend I expected called a few minutes ago. He won't be able to make it after all."

"Too bad." Jeremy glanced at his watch. "Sure, I'll have a glass. No use to waste good sangria. Give me a minute to put my stuff inside and turn on the air conditioning."

The middle son of a long established New Orleans family, Henry Valadon was a junior associate in a busy law firm. Immigration Law was his specialty. Dark brown, wavy hair and smooth, pale olive skin set off his classical good looks and marked him as a Creole descendent. His tight, trim body could only have resulted from regular exercise.

Taking up residence in the French Quarter was one of the ways Henry distanced himself from his close-knit family. He was gay in the quiet, self-confident way of a number of young professionals. He had tested HIV-negative, though some of his friends had not. Jeremy and Joe had made it possible for Henry to keep his friends up to date in the battle against AIDS.

Jeremy walked to the rear of the courtyard and unlocked his apartment, a single large room with an adjoining bathroom and one closet. Once living quarters for household slaves, it had been renovated as an efficiency apartment. A compact kitchen was hidden by louvered folding doors, and a large sofa bed allowed the room to be either a living room or a bedroom. They'd used colorful throw rugs to cover much of the old brick floor.

The slave-quarters apartment suited Jeremy and Joe, since neither of them had time to care for a larger place and only rarely were they both there on the same night. Both of them enjoyed intelligent conversation with someone outside the confining world of medicine, and their friendship with Henry Valadon had grown into a bond of mutual confidence.

When Jeremy returned to the courtyard, Henry had added a tray of cheese and fresh fruit to the table. "I'm ready for the sangria, Henry, but I'll pass on the snacks. I have a dinner date tonight."

Henry poured cold sangria from the ceramic pitcher into a second glass. "I'm sorry to hear that. I was hoping we could have a long evening of conversation." He spread a dollop of warm Brie on a cracker. "Who are you going out with? Anybody I know?"

"Barbara Allison. Do you know her? She's a nurse at the hospital—works on one of the medical wards." Jeremy grinned, then glanced around and lowered his voice in mock secrecy. "Barbara's a pretty foxy lady. I hope I can convince her to stay here tonight."

Henry smiled. "Yeah, I remember Barbara. You brought her to my Christmas party last year. She's a looker, all right. Where are you having dinner?"

Jeremy told him the evening's plans, and Henry nodded his approval. After a long sip of sangria he asked, "Anything new going on at the research lab?"

"There is something new. I don't know much about it yet, but our chief thinks it may be the breakthrough we've all been waiting for. I should learn more next week—I have a clearance to tour the lab on Thursday. I'll keep you posted."

"Please do." Henry stirred the sangria and shook his head. "Man, I hope your chief is right. We need a breakthrough. Some of my friends live every day of their lives in fear of developing AIDS before a real cure comes along."

"So do other people. Henry. A lot of other people."

The attorney leaned forward and looked intently at Jeremy. A little smile teased the corners of his eyes. "Some of my friends think you're gay, you know." He waited in silence for a few seconds, but Jeremy said nothing. "They all know I'm HIV-negative, and they assume you're positive since you work at Charity—can I still call it Charity?"

Jeremy nodded and Henry let out an awkward laugh. "So... they've concluded you and I are probably not having an affair. One or two of 'em would kill for a chance to get to know you a little better."

Jeremy felt heat rise in his face. He tried to laugh, but it didn't come out right. "Your friends are nice people, Henry, but no thanks. No offense intended—just tell 'em I'm not gay."

His words triggered recollection of a long-forgotten experience. He smiled and propped his feet on the edge of the fountain. "For a while though, back when I was in high school, I thought I might be gay."

A cough interrupted Henry's drinking. He put his glass down on the table. "What do you mean, thought?"

"Nothing really. I fell in love with another boy and I thought that meant I was gay. It was my first year of swimming, and I had a big crush on a senior who was captain of the boys' team. Great looking guy. President of his class, an incredible swimmer. I spent a lot of time in the locker room that year, just hoping he'd notice me and feel some of the same things I felt."

Henry refilled both of their glasses. "For God's sake, Jeremy, don't stop now. What happened? Did he ever notice you?"

"Yes, he did. He noticed me from the very beginning. He avoided me for as long as he could, then he made damn sure our friendship stayed casual and proper. At the end of that year, after he graduated, he turned down a swimming scholarship at the University of Texas. Went to New York instead…to study theater.

"I heard later he was doing pretty well. A few roles off Broadway, bit parts in some bigger shows. His family told me he was beginning to attract the attention of major producers. Then, about six years after he left Beaumont, he died of AIDS. After he died his sister told me he was gay—she was the only one in the family who knew it. I really believe I would have gone anywhere with that guy if he'd given me the slightest encouragement." Jeremy shrugged and looked at Henry. "After that, I never had another gay inclination."

"What a story. He never made a sexual approach?"

"He deliberately avoided it. He was sure in my fantasies, but that was it." After a long pause Jeremy looked up sheepishly. "I haven't told many people about that, Henry. I'd rather you didn't spread it around."

"My lips are sealed, friend." Henry took a swallow of sangria, then said. "Hearing you tell that story makes it easy to understand why you're such a thoughtful guy."

"Don't overdramatize it, Henry. I'm sure lots of people have experiences like that."

Henry shook his head. "I don't think so. For sure, nothing like that ever happened to me. If it had, I'd probably still be living in New York—AIDS and all."

The distant clock in the spire of St. Louis Cathedral struck six-thirty, and Jeremy drained his glass. "I better get going. I'm meeting Barbara at eight."

After a long, hot shower and the day's second shave, he lay down on the sofa to cool off in the air conditioned room. How did anybody survive around here before air conditioning? The heat was bad enough, but this damn humidity must have made dressing for the evening a sporty course in the old days.

13

Barbara

Jeremy's father had given him a Miata MX-5 when he graduated from medical school—a metallic silver, two-seated roadster with black leather interior and a convertible top. He loved that car and thought it must have been made for nights like this one promised to be. As a final touch, he folded the soft top down before leaving to meet Barbara for cocktails at the Meridien Hotel. When he pulled out of his parking space to drive the few blocks to Canal Street, he could still feel the mystique of the Quarter, now magnified by the warm glow of late summer dusk. Nightfall came fast and, by the time he left the car with the Meridien's valet, Canal Street was blazing with street lamps.

After drinks he planned to drive uptown for dinner at a small restaurant in one of the old houses on tree-lined St. Charles Avenue. Few tourists knew of the place, but it was popular among locals and a Friday night reservation had taken two weeks' notice. Hopefully, everything was in place to make this a very special night.

Then Barbara walked into the lounge at the Meridien, and he knew for certain it would be a special night. She was breathtaking in a sheer, pale yellow, long-sleeved outfit that perfectly complemented her trim figure, her auburn hair and brown eyes. He stood and held out his hands to her. "You look fantastic," he said. When he leaned to kiss her on the cheek he caught a whiff of her subtle fragrance and grinned. "You smell pretty good, too."

"Thank you, kind sir." She stepped back and beamed. "You don't look too bad yourself. We should get out of hospital whites more often."

The waiter brought the scotch Jeremy had ordered. "What would you like, Barbara?"

She smiled at him and glanced at the waiter. "Chablis-Cassis, please."

"Thanks for meeting me here," Jeremy said.

"Don't thank me for that. It's much more sensible than your coming all the way out to my apartment. I know something about your work schedule, remember?"

"Well, it's very nice of you anyway." His eyes moved over her body. "I've missed seeing you for the past few days. How's your week going?"

"Busy. You know the cardiology ward. And my new job takes a lot of time making out schedules, managing the unit, and all that."

"That's right—you've started as day shift charge nurse."

She nodded. "Day before yesterday."

"That's great, Barb. Congratulations."

"Thanks...I'd rather spend more time taking care of the patients, but it's a good career move." She smiled. "Anyway, I'm glad I have the next couple of days off. We've had three unexpected deaths on the ward this week."

Jeremy urged her away from shop talk and, after the drinks, they retrieved the Miata and drove uptown on St. Charles Avenue. Steering around Lee Circle, the wheels of the small car jumped in and out of some of the city's last remaining streetcar tracks.

They left the Miata with a uniformed attendant in the porte-cochere of an old mansion near First Street, then walked through a small garden to the front door of the house. Jeremy rang the bell and a butler in white tie answered immediately. He bowed graciously and showed them into a Victorian parlor; rose damask covered the walls, richly upholstered sofas and love seats were placed alongside small wooden tables with lamps. As soon as they sat a server appeared with crystal glasses of Pouilly-Fuissé on a small silver tray. The restaurant had a single seating each evening, and its fixed menu changed daily according to the early morning availability of fresh ingredients at the French Market.

A short time later they were seated in a small, elegant dining room where they began their dinner with the house specialty, an exquisitely presented artichoke and oyster appetizer served on fine China. Jeremy winked. "What do you think, Barb? Shall we try the whole dinner?"

Barbara laughed quietly and touched his hand. "It's wonderful, silly. Thank you for choosing this place. I've wanted to come here for a long time."

The night's entree was pompano, stuffed with spicy crab meat and baked *en papillote*. With that course, the servers poured an Alsatian Gewürztraminer. During dinner Barbara and Jeremy's talk wandered back to medicine. He remembered how his mother used to complain about that and he felt a twinge of guilt, but he continued anyway. "Tell me about those unexpected deaths on your ward."

Barbara touched her napkin to the corners of her mouth, then said, "The deaths took us by surprise, Jeremy. Each one was a man in his forties or fifties recovering from an uncomplicated heart attack. They were all within days of going home." She looked at Jeremy and shook her head. "The second one had already started cardiac rehab."

"What happened to them? New heart problems?"

"No. It was more like sepsis or something."

"Like an overwhelming infection?"

She nodded. "High fever. Borderline shock. Mental confusion."

Puzzled, Jeremy frowned. Sounded odd—three in a row like that.

"They'd all been doing well," Barbara said. "The night nurse told us they were fine when the lab technologist came by sometime after midnight to draw blood. It was the same for all three. After that they started to go bad, for no apparent reason. The doctors tried everything." Barbara shrugged in frustration. "Nothing made any difference. Each one of 'em died a few hours after it started. One on Wednesday morning, two yesterday. The whole unit is demoralized."

Jeremy wanted to share her concern, felt like he ought to, but he didn't know exactly what to say. "I'm sure the residents are demoralized. Presenting unexplained deaths at staff conference can be rough."

"They always present the deaths, Jeremy. That's nothing new."

"Sure, but you know how death conferences go. The staff always presume something more, or something different, could have been done to save the patients. Their questions go after it, whatever it is, like a prosecuting attorney, and the residents have to defend their management of the patients. It's like being on trial or something—only you're guilty until you convince everybody in the room otherwise."

"I do know it's like that, but it seems unfair in these cases. Nothing more could have been done for any of them. Nothing different."

Jeremy looked at Barbara and felt a rush of emotion. She was in her milieu in this place—her own elegant beauty enhanced the richness of the dining room. He felt proud that even the servers seemed to take special notice of her. He reached across the table and took her hand. "Hey, that's enough hospital stuff. We have better things to talk about tonight."

Dinner ended with a small serving of strawberries in orange liqueur with freshly whipped cream and a demitasse of dark-roasted espresso. Driving back downtown, Jeremy crossed Canal Street then deliberately avoided the touristy streets in the Quarter, choosing instead the romantic ambiance of gas-lighted Jackson Square and the French Market.

The powerful aroma of New Orleans coffee and fresh beignets filled the air when Jeremy pulled the Miata into a parking space near the Café du Monde. Glancing at Barbara, he reconsidered the idea of more food and winked instead. "Let's take a walk along the levee. It should be nice tonight, warm as it is."

She smiled and touched his arm. "I'd love it."

They walked up the stairs to a boardwalk atop the levee. Higher than the surrounding area, that view enhanced the shadowy intrigue of the busy harbor and the Port of New Orleans. A deep-throated horn interrupted the sound of boats moving through the muddy waters of the Mississippi River. Fishy smells drifted up from the waterfront. Lights of the West Bank twinkled across the broad waterway and added yet another dimension to the romance of the night. Jeremy hugged Barbara close to shelter her from the cool wind blowing up from the river. He wanted to shout with joy when she pressed even closer.

When they returned to the car Jeremy drove past the French Market to Ursulines Avenue. When he downshifted for the turn, Barbara touched his hand. "The Quarter really is beautiful at night isn't it?"

A few blocks later, when he turned onto Burgundy Street, Jeremy took her hand in his. No words were necessary when he parked the car a short block from the apartment. He sensed an unspoken agreement that she was coming in.

In the flickering glow of the courtyard's gaslight, Jeremy slipped his arm around Barbara's waist. "Let's have a liqueur out here by the fountain."

Barbara nodded. "Nothing sweet for me, please. I'd prefer a brandy, if you have it, but first I need the little girls room."

Jeremy showed her into the apartment then busied himself with fixing the drinks. A fleeting thought nagged at him, something she'd said at dinner. Something was out of place in what she had told him about the deaths on her ward, something not quite right. He couldn't figure out exactly what it was, but it was stuck in the back of his mind.

When Barbara returned she had removed the sheer jacket that covered her sleeveless dress. On the patio she sat close to Jeremy. He smelled her fragrance again, like magnolia blossoms on a spring night. The sounds of the splashing fountain combined playfully with a few bars of jazz that floated through the courtyard from some nearby club. Passing footsteps on the cobblestones, then distant laughter joined the medley to create the seductive night music of the French Quarter.

Their hands touched as they sipped the drinks. It felt so right, like the most natural thing in the world when she said, "Jeremy, I want to stay here tonight."

Time stood still for Jeremy. His response had to be precisely right, not the howl of joy that he felt, not the grateful scream that was growing inside him. Restraining himself, he stood and drew her into his arms. "And I want you to stay, Barbara. I want that with all my heart." He kissed her, gently at first, then with barely controlled passion. "But, you know we can't risk pregnancy."

She looked up into his eyes. "Not a problem…I started the pill."

Jeremy smiled, hoping his own eyes expressed physical desire as eloquently as hers. He held her tightly against his body and felt goose flesh rising on her arms. He kissed her again, her lips, her neck.

He was embarrassed to realize he'd been joking around way too much about getting Barbara in the sack. How different it was, now that it was actually happening. He wanted to celebrate it with dignity, like a sacrament. He longed to worship her body, explore her lips, her neck, the soft flesh of her breasts. He ached to consume her and be consumed by her. They stood together in close embrace for a long moment then, without words, walked hand-in-hand into Jeremy's apartment.

He closed the door. Flickering light from the courtyard gaslights enhanced the seductive ambiance of the room. Barbara kissed him gently then turned toward the window. "I love the soft light dancing through the leaves."

The need for her touch pulled him after her. He slid his arms around her from behind and she snuggled back into him. He moved his hands to her breasts. Her hands covered his, then she offered her neck for his kisses.

She gasped when his lips caressed her ear. "Jeremy."

His name had never sounded so wonderful. Her body caressed his as she turned in his arms. He struggled for control. Her eyes held him, burning into the core of him, as she slowly unbuttoned his shirt. Her fingertips, so gentle, combed through the thatch of blond hair on his chest, then teased his nipples. Could she feel his heart pounding?

"Barbara." It was a prayer. He kissed her. Again. Then again. Urgently now, she pulled his shirt from his trousers. Her dress fluttered to the floor and with a quick motion she slipped out of her underthings. God, she was beautiful. "Barbara," he whispered. His hand stroked the satin of her breast. Then the other one, now both. Driven, he had to have more—he tore off the rest of his clothes.

She trembled when his moist tongue flirted with her nipple. "Take me, Jeremy," she begged. "Take me now."

The growing heat inside him flared into a raging inferno and he moved the two of them to the bed. Intensity became urgency. She moaned as his kisses explored her body. Then, in a single graceful movement, she rolled over on top of him and drew him inside her.

Together they moved to the primal cadence of joined lovers. Slowly at first, then with rising crescendo as the two became one. He struggled to hold back until they could both fly through the flames of explosive orgasms.

For a long time they lay silent, still entwined. When they parted, he kissed her lips softly and slipped his arm across her belly. "I love you, Barbara."

Her deep, regular breathing comforted Jeremy as he drifted toward sleep, but his innermost thoughts were disturbing. This intimacy with Barbara was beautiful. The special warmth. The glow. The close solitude they shared. Together, yet apart from everything else. He wanted to capture it forever, make it their own special sacrament. Yet marriage seemed hopeless—there could never be children until there was a way to get the HIV out of their bodies. And what about each other? Did they have the same viral strain? Did they risk doubly infecting each other?

❖❖❖

14

SURGERY STAFF CONFERENCE

JEREMY WOKE EARLY THE NEXT MORNING. DAYBREAK FLOODED THE room with soft light and painted Barbara's sleeping form with an alabaster glow. She was beautiful. So still, sleeping like a baby. What he really wanted was to crawl back under the covers with her, to hold her again. But it was too late for that, he was obligated to make rounds with his junior residents before the weekly staff conference.

He stayed quiet as he put on running clothes, knowing there'd be plenty of time to shower and dress at the hospital. He slipped his wallet into the hip pocket of his shorts—he'd need that damned HIV card to get through the M-E-P. He put his car keys next to the coffee pot and sat at the small table to write a note:

> Barbara, Good morning. Wonderful evening! Wonderful girl! Thanks with all my heart. Please drive yourself home and meet me at the hospital for lunch on Sunday. I should be able to get away around noon. Coffee and fixings—and the car keys—are in the kitchen. I love you.
>
> J…

Outside, he felt good, running through the morning air…it persisted as his favorite time of day. The Saturday streets in the Quarter were especially quiet and his mind wandered among his new feelings of responsibility toward Barbara and toward their relationship. In twenty minutes Big Charity came into view as he turned the corner a block short of it. He remembered Joe would be presenting his post-operative patient's unexpected death at the morning's conference.

Jeremy easily negotiated the M-E-P and took an elevator directly to his fourteenth floor room. After a fast shower and shave, he had just enough time for a quick breakfast before he joined his team for morning rounds. All of their patients were doing well, and Jeremy was especially pleased to find his own Mrs. LeCompte sitting up, eating breakfast.

When she saw him with the group she beamed. "Morning, Dr. Becker. I feel good today, real good. When are you gonna let me go home?"

"You keep on doing this well and it won't be much longer. Maybe another three or four days, okay?"

The rounds took less time than usual, and Jeremy arrived early at the Delgado Amphitheater. He spotted his roommate on the lower level shuffling through a large stack of x-rays.

"Morning, Joe. Do you have everything you need?"

"I hope so, my case is first on the agenda. I think I'm all set—except for one thing. I still don't know why Mr. Gilmore died. The autopsy didn't show anything unexpected. "He waved his hand in helpless frustration. "Even that final blood culture was negative."

Joe continually arranged and rearranged the same stack of x-rays. "Dr. Reynolds is pretty upset. I bet he's gonna eat my team alive this morning."

Jeremy took the x-rays from him and arranged them in chronological order. "Calm down, Joe. The Chief won't let Reynolds be too hard on you. He'll know you couldn't have done anything more to keep Mr. Gilmore from dying."

"Okay, thanks, Jeremy. I'll try to relax." His shoulders drooped. He appeared calm, but he stayed quiet, brooding.

"Listen," Jeremy said, "I still want to help. Let me describe my findings from the night before your patient died. He was doing so well when I saw him."

"Well...okay, Jeremy. I'll go along with that, if you still want to do it. Maybe it'll help the presentation. It'll make me feel better, anyway."

It was time to begin, and Joe took a seat on the lower level with the other residents scheduled to present cases. The entire surgical staff and a large group of medical students filled the amphitheater. Custom reserved the first row for the attending staff, with the Chief always seated at the exact center. Every seat in the amphitheater was filled.

To Jeremy, sitting on the lower level with all the nervous presenters, the audience appeared to crush in from all sides like cynical Roman citizens waiting for a kill in the coliseum. He identified the attendees by the coats they wore: suit coats for the attending staff, long white coats for residents, short white coats for interns, beige coats for medical students. Senior members of the medical faculty held special M-E-P passes that allowed limited entry to the medical center regardless of their HIV status. Each of them in their own way appeared ready to attack the presenters, to find some flaw in the patient care they were about to describe. An ominous hush fell over the room when the Chief took his seat.

After opening announcements by the chief resident, it was Joe's turn. He stood like a proud gladiator and related Mr. Gilmore's history. All of his symptoms were common to many patients with rectal cancer. Joe discussed the proctoscopic biopsy and other studies he'd performed to prove the diagnosis. He described each of the x-rays as he displayed them on a large view box.

Turning to face the Chief, he summarized the operation he and Dr. Reynolds had performed to remove the cancer. "When we finished, we thought we'd gotten all of the tumor. We were confident the patient had an excellent chance for permanent cure."

From the first row, Dr. Reynolds nodded his agreement. Joe looked relieved. He glanced at Jeremy, then described the man's slow progress for several days following the operation. "Dr. Becker examined this patient a few hours before his death. I'd like to ask him to present his findings before I continue."

The Chief agreed to the unusual presentation, and Jeremy stood before the group. "My team was on call the night before Mr. Gilmore died. I knew he'd been having problems, so I made a point of seeing him late that night. I examined him at two AM, about six hours before he died. He had improved significantly at that time." Jeremy described his findings, and several of the attending staff nodded agreement that the patient's condition sounded like definite improvement. Dr. Reynolds had a few specific questions, which Jeremy answered to his satisfaction.

Joe continued, "About two hours after Dr. Becker examined Mr. Gilmore, a lab technologist came by to draw a blood culture. The nurse on duty knew the patient was better. She told me he'd been sleeping soundly for the first time since his operation, and she didn't want to awaken him, so she sent the technologist away—delayed the blood culture for a couple of hours. That culture later proved to be negative, but shortly after the technologist drew the blood—"

Jeremy jumped to his feet, interrupting the presentation. He suddenly realized exactly what Joe had said. "Who did you say drew the blood for that culture?"

The outburst startled Joe. He acted annoyed. "I don't know exactly who it was. The nurses said it was a lab tech. What difference does it make who drew the blood?"

Dr. Reynolds held up his hand to end the confusing discussion. "Sit down, Becker. It doesn't matter who drew the blood culture. Go on with your presentation, Dr. Monteleone."

Jeremy remained standing. "Sir, I believe it does matter. Something is not right here. The laboratory is way too short of technologists to have one of them drawing blood on the wards in the middle of the night, and the nurses are not allowed to do it. Blood samples collected outside the laboratory are practically always drawn by the interns or medical students. No one on my team was in the ICU after I examined Mr. Gilmore. We didn't draw that blood culture, Dr. Reynolds, and I can't buy the notion that a lab tech just happened to be available for a change. I don't know what's going on, sir, but something is not right."

Scraps of conversation ran through the amphitheater.

"He's right. My ward can never get a lab tech."

"Mine, either. I always have to draw the blood."

"The ICU calls us to draw blood for my team."

One of the interns said, "I was in the house that night. Nobody called me to draw a blood culture."

Jeremy stayed quiet, but he tried to remember exactly what Joe had told him on the morning Gilmore died. Yes, he did say a technologist drew that blood culture. It didn't make any sense. Whoa, Barbara had told him something about blood drawing on her patients, too—the three who died. Did she mention who drew their blood?

Comments and discussions around the amphitheater grew louder until, finally, the Chief restored order. "You're right about the shortage of technologists, Dr. Becker, but everyone here knows you may be more sensitive than most of us to issues of blood drawing. "He flashed a condescending smile toward Jeremy. "I'm sure there's a logical explanation for a technologist being in the ICU that night. I'll ask the laboratory chief about it, maybe he can clear up the mystery for you. "He turned toward Joe. "Dr. Monteleone, was this patient enrolled in the AIDS testing program?"

Joe flipped through the pages of his patient's record before he answered. "Yes sir, he was enrolled, but he hadn't received any of the experimental treatments because of his post-op fever. His screening blood counts showed normal T-cells, normal WBC. He was a candidate for the treatment group, but he had fever constantly until that night before his death. When Dr. Becker examined him, his temp was normal for the first time."

Joe completed his presentation, describing the final hours of Gilmore's life A pathology resident presented the autopsy findings, projecting microscopic slides prepared from the patient's organs and tissues. Abnormal findings were limited to those caused by the recent operation. Satisfactory healing was present, and no evidence of cancer remained. The post-mortem examination did not demonstrate a cause for Mr. Gilmore's death.

The staff concluded the patient had died as a result of some undetected infection. None of them acted completely satisfied with that unscientific conclusion, but no one had a better suggestion.

The conference continued for another hour and a half. The group discussed several other patients, but Jeremy was never able to shake off the feeling Joe's case had brought on, a feeling of unfinished business. Afterward, he helped Joe gather up the x-rays and charts, and the two of them stopped in the surgeons' lounge for a cup of coffee.

Relaxed, now, Joe said, "Why are you so upset about the blood drawing business in the Gilmore case? The Chief must have thought you'd gone off the deep end."

"I know. I'm sorry I caused so much commotion."

"Dr. Reynolds didn't know what you were talking about. Neither do I, Jeremy. Maybe the Chief's right—maybe you have gone off the deep end."

"I told you I'm sorry, Joe. I don't know exactly what it's about either. It may have something to do with recent deaths on the medicine ward Barbara told me about."

"What does that have to do with my patient? You really are acting crazy. What did Barbara do to you last night anyway?"

"Forget it, Joe. Maybe it's nothing. I'll check around and get better info. If it makes more sense then, I'll tell you about it. Meanwhile, can you just let it go?"

"Hey, okay. Whatever you say. It's just that I've just never seen you so worked up over the death of a patient who didn't even belong to your team."

Jeremy refilled his coffee cup. "Listen, you better get going. Your day off is slipping away fast. Do you want me to look at any of your patients tonight?"

Joe laughed. No, thanks. I get in trouble when you do that."

"Come on, Joe. I'm serious."

"No, everybody's stable. The junior residents can let you know if anything changes."

"By the way," Jeremy said, "I didn't have time to straighten up the apartment this morning. Sorry about that. I'll owe you a house cleaning."

"Don't worry about it, it's not important. I don't have any special plans for today anyway."

❖ ❖ ❖

15

LENNIE'S SECRET

BY THE TIME HE WAS TWELVE YEARS OLD LENNIE WAS STAYING one or two nights every week at Miss Rena's house. Once he got used to being around that stone lady, she wasn't so bad. She smelled funny, kind of flowery, but she was good to him all the time. Told him stories about how things used to be in Thibodaux. She made sure Lucifer bought things Lennie liked when he went to the store and she told the cook special ways to fix 'em. She always had a peach pie or a chocolate cake or something like that when he spent the night.

She wasn't really turning to stone. Lucifer told him she'd had some kind of sickness when she was a little girl, so now she couldn't move her legs right. That's why he helped her in and out of the car. She used a rolling chair in the house, and she even let Lennie try it out one day. She laughed a lot, too. Lennie wasn't used to that—grownups laughing around the house—but he liked it. It made him feel good.

The nights he stayed would usually be just before or right after Mr. Marshall's regular Thursdays in Thibodaux. Sometimes Mr. Marshall would spend the night, too. He wanted the two of 'em to spend more time together, he told Lennie, so they could talk about things.

They did talk a lot. Lennie had never talked much to a grown man and he knew he had a lot to learn. Talking was one thing his daddy never had done much of, so he took pleasure in just about anything Mr. Marshall wanted to talk about.

That was the year his mama died, the year after Lennie was twelve. Cancer they said. Mr. Marshall took care of everything, gave her a nice burial and moved Lennie into Miss Rena's house full time.

Lennie finally got up the nerve one day to stop calling his benefactor

Mr. Boudreaux or Mr. Marshall. That was just about that same time Marshall started to change, too. He still looked after Lennie, all right. Bought him clothes and things. And he kept on paying Lennie for his work at Miss Rena's, even took him to the bank one day to open a savings account for most of the money. But, around that time, he started finding more and more things for Lennie to do, hard things. Scrub the big front porch every week, paint the screens, clean out the garage, dig up the garden, things like that.

In other ways Marshall got mean. He told Lennie things that made him believe it was his own fault Mama died. "She had a hard birth with you," Marshall said. "You came out feet first and tore her up inside. She lost an awful lot of blood, almost died right then. Never could have any more babies. That's probably why she got that cancer."

Lennie worried about that. He sure didn't mean to kill his mama. He didn't remember doing it. He didn't want her to die. She was the only person he'd ever loved. Now Daddy, he was something different. He was bad. Mean as a rattlesnake, nothing good about that man. He deserved what happened to him. But not Mama, she was a good woman.

Later that year Marshall started taking Lennie to New Orleans with him for holidays, sometimes even for regular weekends. Lennie was pretty scared the first time. It was fifty-some miles in Marshall's big Lincoln—longest trip he'd ever made.

Miss Rena had told him Marshall's wife was uppity. A New Orleans society woman, she'd said, out to get Marshall's money. She never came to Thibodaux, so he didn't meet her at all until he got to their house in Metairie.

Well, Metairie was a rich folks' neighborhood all right, but Lennie liked Marshall's wife. They didn't have any children of their own and she was real nice to him. She made a special room for him in their house—Lennie's room, she called it. Said he could go in there and close the door any time he wanted to. Sometimes, when Marshall went to work, she took him for long walks in City Park or out at the lakefront. He liked the lakefront, especially when you could see the sailboats. She even took him over by the Mississippi River and showed him that big ol' bridge goin' across to the West Bank. One day she took him to the zoo, and that was a lot of fun—seein' all those animals from Africa and everywhere.

One of the times in Metairie, Marshall got home late at night and came in Lennie's room to see if he was asleep. He was still awake, so Marshall turned on a dim light. Said he wanted to talk for a while and sat down on the edge of Lennie's bed. They talked about a lot of things. Man things, mostly. What men and women do together, things like that. Then, all at once, Marshall sat up straight and said, “Lennie, I know all about you and your daddy.”

“What do you mean? What about me and my daddy?”

“I know what he did to you. In the shed...?”

“He didn’t do nothing to me, unless you mean the whippin’. He beat the tar outa me sometimes. Had my butt bleedin’ once or twice.”

“That’s not what I mean.”

Lennie looked right at Marshall, but he didn’t say anything.

“You know what I’m talking about. Why don’t you tell me about it?”

Lennie knew all right, but he couldn’t talk about it. Not that. Especially not with Marshall. What if he wanted to do it, too? “I tell you my daddy didn’t do nothin’ to me. I don’t even know what you’re talking about.”

“I think you do know, Lennie. The sheriff told me your clothes were practically torn off you. Blood all over you, he said. Shit, too.”

Lennie wanted to cry, but he couldn’t cry and think about his daddy at the same time. Nothing about that man to cry over. “My daddy didn’t do that to me. It was that hobo...the hobo that ran away. I told the sheriff about that.”

“The hobo didn’t leave any tracks in the mud around that shed, Lennie. The posse searched all the way over to the bayou and never found a single sign of any hobo.”

“They didn’t look ’til the next day. That hobo probably stole somebody’s pirogue and got away in the middle of the night.”

“The sheriff found your daddy with his head split open, just like you said, Lennie. But he found something else, too. Your daddy’s pants were unzipped.”

“He didn’t do that. That hobo must have unzipped ’em after he finished with me. I saw him hittin’ my daddy in the head some more—no tellin’ what else he did. Daddy wasn’t moving at all by then, but the hobo picked up the ax handle and tore into him all over again.” Lennie forgot for a minute—was he supposed to know about the ax handle?

Marshall said, “You and I both know there was no hobo that day, Lennie. Your daddy unzipped his own pants, didn’t he? The sheriff figured that, too. He found your daddy with his pecker hanging out.”

Lennie couldn’t talk about it. He was scared. No more words would come out.

“The sheriff left that part out of his report. He’s my brother-in-law, you know. We talked about it, but I convinced him there was no use to write up that part.” He reached under the covers and took Lennie’s hand. “I think it was you, Lennie. You hit your daddy with the ax handle. He probably deserved it, but you did it, didn't you? You killed him."

Tears exploded out of Lennie like a raging cataract. Held back way too long, the tears ran down his face like an untamed river. Marshall lifted him up from the pillow and held him in his arms. Held him tight. Safe, Lennie thought. Finally safe.

❖ ❖ ❖

16

Unexpected Events

After the Saturday morning staff conference Jeremy spent most of the afternoon reviewing the progress of his team's ICU patients and catching up on his medical records. Seemed like he always had medical records that needed one thing or another—a signature here, a dictation there, countersigning a medical student's notes, things like that. He was about ready to go to the staff dining room for supper when one of the junior residents paged him for the Emergency Room. He wanted Jeremy's consultation about a new patient he thought had appendicitis.

The patient turned out to be a young man by the name of Jeff Thompson, a good looking guy in his mid-twenties. He was an athletic type with yellow hair that demanded notice—it was like a golden field of ripe wheat that contrasted sharply with his striking suntan and his deep blue eyes. After asking only a few questions, Jeremy concluded this patient was a little more well-spoken than Charity's usual emergency room clientele.

The man's intense suntan intrigued Jeremy. Smooth and even, it covered his entire body, interrupted nowhere by white swim suit lines—not even a bikini line. Jeremy was curious, but he couldn't think of a diplomatic way to ask the patient about his head-to-toe suntan. Curiosity aside, he agreed with the junior resident's diagnosis and they arranged to admit Thompson to the hospital, with an appendectomy scheduled an hour or two later. Jeremy consulted his attending staff by telephone, and the older man agreed the residents should proceed with an appendectomy, Jeremy assisting Patrick, the junior resident. He cautioned they should call him again if they needed him for any reason.

Then, at supper, Patrick solved the riddle of Thompson's suntan. "Yeah, I noticed it, too," he said. "By the way, I asked about his family. His father's a surgeon in upstate New York."

The intern scratched his head. "What in the world does that have to do with his suntan?"

"Nothing at all. But Jeff's a grad student in archeology, and he just finished a summer semester in Spain."

Jeremy smiled. "Spain? He must have majored in nude beaches."

That started the whole team laughing, and Jeff Thompson instantly became their most famous patient. After Spain, his homeward travel had included a vacation in New Orleans, and when he became ill, he was directed to the HIV-positive hospital. After Jeremy's joke, and especially after learning Thompson was a graduate student and a surgeon's son, the team adopted him as one of their own. Every one of them took a special interest in his well-being.

On his way to the operating room Jeremy stopped by the ward to check on Mrs. LeCompte. Her husband was visiting. Jeremy had learned to recognize their kind of marriage among south Louisiana's Cajun folks. He knew the woman represented everything good in her husband's life. To him she was wife and mother, helpmate and teacher, companion and goddess. She doted on him, and she had absolutely mastered a skill prevalent among women of that culture, a knack for allowing their men to remain in charge, while they themselves actually controlled the destiny of their families.

"Good evening, Mrs. LeCompte. How're you doing tonight? "He shook hands with her husband. "Mr. LeCompte."

The patient answered for both of them. "We're fine, doctor." She hesitated, then said, "My husband was wondering when I'm gonna be ready to go home...so he can make plans for the children, you know."

Jeremy smiled as he flipped through the pages of her chart. She was determined to pin him down. Pretty sly, putting the blame on her husband. "Well, let's see. No fever. None since the first day after your operation. Everything else looks good. Let's plan for you to leave about Wednesday, okay? That'll be exactly a week after your operation."

LeCompte grinned and smoothed a wrinkle from the sheet on his wife's bed. "That's fine, doctor. We did miss her at home, I guarantee. For sure I'm gonna took good care of her."

"I know you will, Mr. LeCompte. We'll plan on Wednesday if she keeps on doing well." He turned to his patient. "I'm glad to see you volunteered for testing one of the HIV treatments. That's important. If we're going to find the best cure for HIV and AIDS we need to test every new hope that comes along."

"Everybody in the hospital has been so nice to me, Dr. Becker. I want to help any way I can. I know it's important." She smiled and took LeCompte's hand. "My husband volunteered, too. Course he's not a hospital patient, but they accepted him anyway."

The Cajun man looked uncomfortable, probably embarrassed to talk about AIDS with his wife present. "You don't had to tell 'im about that," he said. "It don't mean nothing."

Jeremy put his hand on the man's shoulder. "Oh yes, it does. It means a lot. Testing new treatments is important for the two of you and for a lot of other people. I'm real proud of you both for volunteering."

Jeremy joined the team in the operating room. After their new patient was anesthetized the residents discovered his total suntan appeared even more startling under the bright surgical lights. Jeremy heard one of the nurses stifle a gasp when she removed the sheet covering Thompson's body to prepare him for the incision.

To make the situation even more difficult to ignore, the patient's penis became fully erect. The intern tried without much success to suppress a snicker. "Don't worry about it," Jeremy told him. "That happens sometimes with the anesthesia."

The student nurse who had the job of scrubbing Thompson's lower abdomen in preparation for an incision was so flustered she could hardly do her work. She bumped the operating table with her scrub tray and spilled disinfecting solutions everywhere. Crimson herself, she tried to clean up the spill and open a new sterile pack of equipment. Her professionalism gone, she looked ready to burst into tears.

Jeremy put a hand on the young girl's shoulder and said, "It's all right." He looked at the intern. "Tom, please prep the patient for us, will you?"

Tom nodded and began to set up the equipment.

The student nurse glanced at Jeremy with grateful brown eyes above her surgical mask. She left the room as quickly as she could. The more experienced circulating nurse whispered, "Thanks, Dr. Becker."

Jeremy managed to get his junior resident into the scrub room before they both burst into laughter. Patrick said, "Jeremy, that young nurse'll be your friend for the rest of her life. She probably never saw an erect penis at close range before."

"She'll be all right."

Patrick had performed only one previous appendectomy. Jeremy shared his thrill at being able to carry out the operation with smooth precision, their four hands working together in a symphony of movement like they were controlled by a single brain. Jeremy told the others about the special pleasure he got when teamwork clicked like that in the operating room. "It happens just often enough to make the drudgery of our residency a little bit easier."

Jeff's appendix was acutely inflamed, but not ruptured, and the residents expected the operation to return him to good health in short order. After completing the appendectomy, the team found the hospital quiet—oddly quiet for a Saturday night. Jeremy made a final pass through the ICU, then went to his room to read an article or two in the latest issue of the American Journal of Surgery. As frequently happened, he fell asleep before he finished the first article.

Shortly after midnight his chance for a solid night's sleep was foiled by a persistent ringing bell. Groggy, he groped for the phone. Damn, he thought, that's the biggest penalty of a surgery residency—the telephone becomes your enemy. "Becker here, what is it?" He instantly recognized the voice of his junior resident, Patrick, the man who'd earlier performed that appendectomy with such skill.

"Dr. Becker, Mrs. LeCompte is having problems."

"What do you mean? What kind of problems?"

"She started to deteriorate about twenty minutes ago—fever spiked to one-oh-three. She still has fever and she's pretty confused right now."

Jeremy could not believe what he was hearing. There had to be some mistake. It couldn't be Mrs. LeCompte—she was fine a few hours ago. He sat up and swung his feet to the floor. "What's her blood pressure? Does her wound look okay?"

"Her pressure's normal—the wound is clean. Her lungs are clear, Jeremy. No leg tenderness, no coughing. I can't find anything wrong but the fever and mental confusion."

"Okay, I'll be right there. Go ahead and send a blood culture and a white cell count. Better get a dose of IV steroids ready, too, but don't give it yet. We can decide about using it when I get there." Ready as Jeremy was for quick response to emergencies, he was not prepared for this turn of events. His mind raced, searching for an explanation.

Minutes after hanging up the telephone he rushed into the ward. Dim lights blurred the large room's size and gave its shape an ominous feeling like some underground cavern. The team had placed portable screens around Mrs. LeCompte's bed, and the nearby goose neck lamps cast huge, eerie shadows on the ceiling. Other patients in the open ward had followed an unspoken rule of hospital courtesy—they had turned away from the stricken patient and pretended to sleep.

Patrick, the intern, two medical students, and a nurse were crowded inside the screens, all working together with organized desperation to keep Mrs. LeCompte alive. Jeremy recognized their seemingly chaotic activity as purposeful. One team member observed and recorded the team's every action. Another was starting a second IV line and drawing blood for the studies Jeremy wanted. They had already inserted a urinary catheter, and a pressure cannula was secured in an artery at the patient's wrist. Adhesive electrodes were attached to her bare chest. Amber lines tracking her blood pressure, pulse and EKG marched endlessly across a bedside monitor's dark video screen, all punctuated by the staccato rhythm of an audible pulse monitor.

Jeremy saw at a glance that the woman's blood pressure was low and her pulse way too rapid. The urine collecting bag was practically empty. Her skin was pale and covered with tiny dew-like droplets of sweat. Her breathing was rapid, and her lips were dusky and bluish-gray despite the oxygen flowing through a green cannula inserted into her nostrils.

This patient who had been so well a few short hours earlier was now in profound shock, struggling to stay alive. The scene reeked of human smells, the pungent smells of human bodies engaged in life or death combat.

Without words, the others made a place at the bedside for Jeremy. He took his patient's hand. Her skin felt warm and clammy—too warm. He leaned close to her ear and spoke softly. "Mrs. LeCompte, it's Dr. Becker. You've got high fever, and we're all working hard to find out why. I'll be right here. We have to do a lot of things in a hurry. If we hurt you, try to let me know. Are you having pain right now? Do you hurt anywhere? Squeeze my hand if you do."

No response. Jeremy turned to the others. "What are her other vital signs? Anything I can't see on the monitor?"

The patient's nurse said, "Her temp's still over a hundred three. We gave her twenty grains of aspirin by rectum. The aide's fixing alcohol and ice right now." Jeremy nodded his agreement. "Her blood pressure's still falling. Eighty-five over fifty right now. Pulse a hundred thirty and weak. You can see her mental state has gotten worse—she's completely unresponsive now."

"I see that. Did she tell you anything before? Anything about how she felt?"

"No, Dr. Becker, she was too confused. Just crying out for her children. I have the steroid injection ready—want me to give it now?"

"Yes. Give it slowly, in the IV line. And keep trying to cool her off. Start sponging as soon as the aide gets here." He parted the screens and stepped out. "I want to talk to the charge nurse for a minute."

Still searching for answers, Jeremy walked to the nearby nurses' station. What had gone wrong? They had to be missing something. What was it—what in the hell was it? How in God's name could he turn things around?

The nurse stood up from the charting desk as Jeremy approached. About fifty, she was someone he knew as one of the more experienced and capable RNs on the staff.

"I'm sorry about this, Dr. Becker. I know she's a special patient for you. She was fine when my shift came on duty." The nurse shrugged and shook her head. "Smiling, feeling good. Vital signs normal. She told us she'd be going home in a few days."

"Thanks, Parrish. She is special." They both sat down, and Jeremy tried to recreate the events leading to his patient's deterioration. He knew a detailed review often focused some faint glimmer of light that revealed a clearer picture. "When did you first suspect she was going bad?

"She got sick just before midnight."

"What was happening at that time?"

"Nothing, really. When the nurse aide made her rounds Mrs. LeCompte asked for a blanket."

"Did she complain of anything? Chest pain or shortness of breath or anything else out of the ordinary?"

Mrs. Parrish shook her head. "No, she said she felt cold and had a little headache. The aide thought that was odd because it's not cold in this ward. She took her temp—it was a hundred and three."

"Nothing else? Just the fever?"

"That's all. Her temp went up fast. The evening shift had checked it with the ten o'clock vitals. It was normal then."

Jeremy glanced toward his patient's bed. "What was she like when you examined her, Parrish? What did you find?"

"I went to check on her as soon as the aide told me about her elevated temp." She opened the patient's chart and pointed to the notes she had written. "She seemed fine except for the fever. Mild headache was her only complaint. No other pain, no difficulty breathing. She wasn't cyanotic at that time, and her mental status was completely clear."

She looked at Jeremy and frowned. "Right then, while I was at the bedside with her, she began to go downhill fast. So fast I called the intern and your junior resident at the same time. When I told them who it was they both got here in a hurry." She shook her head. "I knew she was in trouble."

Jeremy was as clueless as ever. He picked up a yellow pencil from the desk and rolled it between his hands. "The evening shift didn't report anything unusual?"

"No, nothing at all. Mrs. Evans was charge nurse on the three to eleven shift. You know how thorough she is."

"Right. I remember seeing Evans when I came by earlier."

"She mentioned you were here. We all knew you had a special interest in this patient." She smiled and patted Jeremy's arm. "Evans told me a lab technologist was here just before shift change. He came to draw the blood culture you asked him to collect. Evans said—"

"What…?" Jeremy jumped up from his chair. For the first time in their conversation, maybe the first time in his life, he yelled at the nurse. "What blood culture, Parrish? I didn't order any blood culture for this patient!"

❖❖❖

17

ANTITHESES

AFTER JEREMY'S OUTBURST, MRS. PARRISH DREW HERSELF upright and folded her hands on the patient's chart. "Evans knew she didn't have an order for any blood work, Dr. Becker. When she spotted the technologist at your patient's bed, she asked him what he was doing. He showed her the request for blood culture with your name on it. He told her you'd called it directly to the lab."

She glanced into the ward and lowered her voice. "Evans told me she thought it was odd to have a blood culture when Mrs. LeCompte was doing so well. But she saw the lab slip, and the technologist had a hospital ID badge, so she let him draw the blood."

For Jeremy, the *dèjá vu* was overpowering. What in the hell was happening here? Pulsating contractions in both cheek muscles clenched his jaw so tight his teeth ached. Frustration gave way to growing anger that pounded in his head like an audible heartbeat. "Who was that lab technologist, Parrish? You said it was a man, didn't you? What time was he here—exactly what time? Did Evans see him draw blood from my patient?"

Mrs. Parrish spoke softly. "Evans did say it was a man, Dr. Becker, but I don't know his name. I'm sure he was here around ten-thirty, but I don't think Evans actually watched him draw the blood." At that moment, Jeremy's struggle to understand what was happening was cut short. Mr. LeCompte appeared at the door.

Relief swept over the man's worried face when he saw Jeremy. "Dr. Becker, you're here mighty late." His relief changed to anguish when he spotted the screens around his wife's bed. "What's wrong? What's happen to my wife?"

Jeremy and the nurse both stood up and walked toward LeCompte. They knew they had to stop him before he ran to her bedside. His frantic eyes searched the ward. "Tell me what's happen."

He gazed upward, toward the heavens. "I'm tired like hell, but I could not sleep in that lounge. I decide to walk down here, and what I'm find? She got all them screen around the bed. I'm saw them screen around dead peoples, Dr. Becker." The man's body sagged, but his powerful hands grabbed Jeremy's arms. "Is my wife dead?"

Jeremy pulled away, then both he and the nurse acted by reflex. Each of them took LeCompte by an arm, one on either side. "No, she's not dead," Jeremy said. "She has fever. The team's working to find out why. She's pretty sick right now, but I believe we'll have the answer soon."

Jeremy raised his eyebrows as a signal to the nurse. "Let Mrs. Parrish take you back to the lounge. I'll be out there to talk to you as soon as I can leave here. It shouldn't be too long."

"I need to see my—"

"Please wait in the lounge, Mr. LeCompte. There's nothing you can do to help her right now. She'd want you to wait in the lounge—do it for her. I'll be there soon."

Still protesting, LeCompte left with Mrs. Parrish. Jeremy joined the others at the patient's bedside.

"She's not improving," the intern said. "Did you come up with anything new?"

The nurse handed Jeremy a lab report with a series of computer printed numbers. "The blood gases are back. They look pretty good, but we can't budge her pressure. It's down to seventy-five by palpation. Her temp's soaring, too."

He saw they'd adjusted the bed to elevate the patient's legs. She was completely naked and the bed was soaked from iced alcohol sponging. Idly covering her groin with one of the wet cloths, Jeremy noticed her skin was still hot to his touch.

"Give her another dose of IV steroids," he said to the nurse. "And get an IV piggyback ready, with two grams of a broad spectrum antibiotic."

"Which broad spectrum?"

Jeremy shrugged. "It's a shot in the dark. Just use whichever one you've got ready to go on the unit."

"That new one okay? Ultrasporin? We just got it in this week."

"Great—that covers anaerobes, too. It's the best choice we've got."

She handed the already prepared syringe of a powerful steroid medication to the intern and left to prepare the antibiotic. Jeremy hoped steroids would give the patient's resistance a jump start. He watched the younger man administer it, a desperate hope of buying some time for her body to take a turn for the better. He put his a hand on the intern's arm. "Thanks for all your help, Tom. Stay here, and watch her vital signs closely. Have the nurse start the Ultrasporin as soon as it's ready, and run it in fast."

He glanced at the medical students. "One of you go through a complete physical again. I want to be sure nothing's changed in the last half hour. I'll be at the desk looking over the nursing notes for the past few shifts." He shook his head and squinted. "I'll take any clue I can find. We've got to be overlooking something."

Joining Jeremy at the desk, the junior resident pulled a crumpled handkerchief from his pocket and wiped oily sweat from his forehead. He sat on the edge of the desk, facing Jeremy. "She's not going to make it, is she?"

"I don't think so, Patrick. And we can't do a damn thing about it. I feel fucking stupid, but I can't figure out anything that would help her."

"Me neither—I don't understand it." The resident looked at Jeremy's face. "Listen, why don't you go upstairs and get some rest. We're doing everything we can. We'll all be right here. I'll call you if anything changes."

"No, I need to be here." He clapped Patrick on the shoulder. "Thanks anyway."

The intern called out from the bedside. "Dr. Becker, rapid V. tach!"

Ventricular tachycardia. Jeremy's mind ran through the long-memorized protocols for treating abnormal heart rhythms: Extremely rapid heartbeat. If untreated, likely to progress to ventricular fibrillation—often fatal.

When Jeremy and Patrick reached the bedside, the intern was already giving an IV injection of lidocaine. The EKG monitor showed no change. Jeremy's fingers probed the patient's neck for a pulse. "Repeat the lidocaine. She still has a weak pulse."

The intern injected the second dose. No effect.

Mrs. Parrish returned, and she joined the team at the bedside. "Mr. LeCompte is really in bad shape," she said. "I couldn't do anything with him. Thank God Mrs. LeCompte's sister and her husband are there, too. That brother-in-law is one of the biggest men I've ever seen—he'll keep LeCompte under control."

Listening with half an ear, Jeremy did not break the team's rhythm. He acknowledged the nurse's report with a nod, at the same time ordering a stronger cardiac stimulant for the patient. The intern injected it into the IV line. No effect. A second dose. Still no effect.

Moments later the rapid EKG pattern of heartbeat degenerated to erratic, disorganized twitching. Ventricular fibrillation, the ineffectual rhythm that Jeremy had hoped to prevent. "V. fib!" he announced. "Bob, begin chest compression. Parrish, put the oxygen line on the Ambu bag and start ventilation." He took the electrical defibrillator paddles from the resuscitation cart and looked at the other nurse. "Charge it up. Unsynchronized shock."

The lethal EKG rhythm continued. "Stand back!" Jeremy positioned the two electrical paddles on the conductor pads the nurse had stuck on either side of the patient's bare chest. He thumbed the discharge button on each paddle, sending a surge of current into the woman's body and through the muscle mass of her heart. Her entire body contracted momentarily, like a brief seizure, but the fibrillating heart rhythm continued without change.

"Resume compression and ventilation. Recharge the paddles, higher output."

He administered a second shock and the erratic EKG pattern changed to a flat line.

"Cardiac standstill. Resume compression and ventilation." The team continued their precisely coordinated actions to feed oxygen into the patient's blood stream and pump it to her body's vital organs. After several minutes her heart had still not resumed its own pumping action, and Jeremy began a systematic series of injections intended to stimulate it. He injected one of them directly into her heart and he tried an external pacemaker for electrical stimulation, but nothing produced any response. The patient's heart had no further spontaneous contractions.

Resuscitation continued for another fifty minutes, team members alternating the physically demanding tasks of chest compression and ventilation so fatigue would not diminish their effectiveness. The straight-line EKG tracing never varied. Nothing indicated life in Mrs. LeCompte's heart. Nothing suggested the faintest hope for coaxing it back to its vital role of life-giving pump.

Jeremy looked around the group, pausing for momentary eye contact with each member of the team. "No response at all," he said. "Any other suggestions? At this point I'll try anything."

The team members all shook their heads.

"Okay. Let's stop." He looked at his watch to note the official time of Mrs. LeCompte's death—2:10 AM. The best efforts of a well-oiled medical team had failed. Death was their enemy, the antithesis of everything the medical professions represented. The enemy had won.

Jeremy watched each member of the team begin, without direction, to carry out the tasks required following a patient's death. They were tasks that each of them performed alone, necessary chores that also allowed time for each one to exorcise anger and frustration and sorrow. Jeremy had the most difficult task of all, explaining it all to the LeCompte family.

As he walked down the dark corridor to the family lounge, he tried without success to understand the things he had to discuss. Entering the room, he found LeCompte huddled alone at the window, staring into the darkness. His brother-in-law and that large man's wife sat nearby. The three of them jumped to their feet and rushed toward Jeremy with a barrage of questions.

"How's she doin'? Did the fever gone?"

"Is she better? Can I go see her now?"

"She ain't dead behind them screen is she?"

"Take them screen away, doc. They make me scared like hell."

Jeremy sensed it was necessary to hold this group of emotional people at bay, to calm them, somehow, in order to make them understand the situation. "Mr. LeCompte, can we sit down on the couch? There are several things I want to tell you."

"What is it, doc? She's dead, ain't she? I knew it. I killed that woman dead with them AIDS. I'm told you I did it."

The others tried to calm LeCompte, but all three voices grew louder and louder, and Jeremy couldn't get a word in. The three of them were consoling and berating each other at the same time, half in English, half in French. Jeremy saw no other option than shouting louder than all of them, "Quiet!"

During the moment of shocked silence that followed, he took LeCompte by the arm and led him forcibly to a couch. The other two began arguing between themselves.

"Mr. LeCompte, your wife was fine during the evening. All of a sudden, around midnight, she developed high fever. My whole team was there. We worked as hard as we could to find the cause of the fever."

The in-laws stopped bickering and moved closer.

"In spite of everything we did, she got worse very rapidly. Finally her heart failed. She's gone now."

"Nooooo! No, God, no! I can't stood that!"

Jeremy held LeCompte's arms. "Easy, man, easy. She was unconscious at the end. She had no pain at any time."

There was a long silence, then a loud outburst of wailing and shouting poured from the three of them. Damn, another antithesis. Not at all what Jeremy expected. He stared, dumbfounded, as the two men grabbed his arms and jerked him to his feet. They both began to beat him on the head and shoulders with their fists.

"*Bâton merdeux!* Shitass! You killed her deader than hell." The noise of their outcry was matched by the cracking sounds of powerful fists striking his body.

"*Petit pine!* You little prick! You did it!"

"I saw them death screen. She was sick like hell, and you had them others in there shootin' her with poison."

Each thud filled Jeremy's head with explosive pain.

"*Espèce de con!* Fuckin' idiot! What kinda doctor are you?"

"Yeah, you dumb shit. A real doctor would not did that."

"I oughta kill you dead, jus' like you kill my woman."

The beating continued. A fusillade of pain followed each blow that struck him. Blood ran into his eyes. He tried to defend himself, but he was no match for the two men. He knew he had to get out of there. Had to get away somehow.

Struggling, he fell to the floor and tried to cover his head. A rapid tattoo of hard blows pounded his back. He rolled away. Crashing fists and kicking feet smashed into his gut, his groin. Pain. Pain everywhere.

Running footsteps penetrated his bewildered brain. Who was coming? He couldn't take much more. He heard a new voice. Angry. Unfamiliar. Between the thundering blows he tried to get up, to get away from the men, but his body wouldn't respond. His brain was thick—he could barely think. The attackers whirled around his head like rogue planets in chaotic orbits.

The pain faded. The noise congealed into a roaring, yellow solid, and Jeremy soared far above the brawl. His confused thoughts constricted into a tight circle of intense white light, then vanished altogether. He collapsed and all was black. Finally, no more pain.

❖ ❖ ❖

18

Weldon

LENNIE GOT SO USED TO STAYIN' WITH THE BOUDREAUX FAMILY in New Orleans he wanted to live there all the time, but Marshall wouldn't let him do it. He told him Miss Rena needed him in Thibodaux. Lennie had figured out he had to do whatever Marshall Boudreaux told him. He tried going against him once or twice, but it didn't work.

If he didn't do exactly what Marshall said, the man would take him aside, take him to some private place, and talk to him. "Don't you ever forget, boy," Marshall would say, "I know your secret. I know what you did with your daddy, and I know what it got you into. I know what you did to him with that ax handle. I know you lied to the sheriff about that hobo."

Marshall got a special look on his face when he talked about that stuff. A wild look that scared Lennie. His lips kind of snarled, and his eyes got real beady-lookin'. Shoot, those eyes bored into Lennie like a pair of hot pokers. "Your secret's safe with me, boy...unless you cross me. But, if you ever do cross me, you'll be in big trouble. You'll get everything that's coming to you, I guarantee. Everything. For killing your daddy and for all the rest of it. Don't you ever forget that."

Lennie never asked him exactly what he meant by "all the rest of it." He couldn't mean the fuckin'—that wasn't his idea, he didn't even want to do it. All the same, he got Marshall's meaning and, after a while, they didn't even have to talk about it. Marshall just gave him that look, and Lennie knew he had to shape up.

He figured he was better off, anyway, if he just listened to Marshall and didn't talk back or anything. Marshall got him everything he needed, everything he wanted, as long as Lennie let him make the rules.

Lennie had learned a lot from Mama about going along, about keeping peace in the family. So, he just went along when Marshall told him he had to stay in school in Thibodaux. "You better keep on making passin' grades, too, you hear. I've got big plans for you, boy. You're going to college." He knew Marshall wanted him to get an education, and he took notice of how Marshall got his way about most things.

School was never easy for Lennie. He liked learning things, but he had to work hard to keep his grades up. His friend, Weldon, did a lot better—he got the top grades in the class. Weldon was real smart even though he stayed busy all the time with football and everything. The year before, in junior high, the girls had started giggling after Weldon all the time, but he didn't pay them no mind. One spring day Lennie asked Weldon to explain something to him, something about algebra. Lennie got hung up every time he thought about all those letters and things taking the place of numbers.

They got together after school and Weldon explained some of the algebra problems to him. Lennie said he understood it, then he started asking a few more questions. Pretty soon Weldon was teaching him everything about algebra. Science, too. He met Weldon after practice two or three times a week and they worked on whatever he was having trouble with. They kept on doing that for a while, meetin' in a secret place behind the gym. Then one day Weldon was late. Real late. When he finally got there he put his bike's kick stand down and slouched over to where Lennie was sittin' on the grass.

"I thought you weren't comin'," Lennie said.

"I can't stay. My ma don't want me study with you no more."

"Why not? My algebra grades are a lot better already. Does she know how much you're helpin' me?"

"She knows it." Weldon didn't sit down. Just shuffled around and stayed out of reach of Lennie's eyes. "She told me you ain't s'posed to need me to get good grades. You're s'posed to do it by yourself."

"What's wrong with helpin' me? Has your ma got something against me? What did you tell her?"

"I didn't tell her nothin'. She said it was somethin' about your daddy."

"My daddy?" So that was it. She knew. She must be afraid of him, afraid of what he'd do to Weldon. "My daddy's dead, Weldon. You know that."

"Shoot, I ain't studyin' no daddy. I told Ma that, but she don't like the idea of us hanging around out here behind the school like we do."

"We can go somewhere else. I'll ask Miss Rena. She'll let us study at her house."

"No sir, not me. I ain't goin' in no stone lady's house."

"Come on, Weldon. She's real nice. Anyway, she's not really a stone lady."

"You told me that, but I don't know...." As soon as everybody at school found out Lennie was living in Miss Rena's house, they'd started calling him the stone lady's boy. Said he was gonna turn to stone, too, if he stayed there too long. That part of it didn't seem to bother Weldon until the idea of actually going to her house came up.

"What about your house?" Lennie said. "I don't mind going over there."

"Too much noise. Ma wouldn't let us do it, anyway."

"How'd she find out we were gettin' together? Did you tell her?"

"I don't tell her shit about what I do. Raymond saw us out here. He told her."

"Your brother, Ray?"

"Yeah. He's an asshole. Tells Ma everything."

"Is he still in school?"

"He's a senior. I'll be glad when the fucker graduates. One year in the same school with him is enough for me."

"I don't ever see Raymond around here. At the hardware store sometimes, but not around school."

"He works every afternoon. Weekends, too. Shit, he's even got me set up to work there next summer."

"If he's a senior, maybe he can help me with my classes."

"That dumb bastard? He'll be lucky to graduate. He couldn't teach a flea how to hop."

"Sounds like you hate your brother."

Weldon drew back and looked at him. "Hate him?" He rubbed his ear for a while, then sat down. "Naw, I don't hate him. He's all right. Him and me are the only boys still at home. Just three girls and us two. The other five are gone. They all call me the baby. Shit, that's what bugs me about Raymond. He acts like he's my daddy."

"Acts like your daddy?" Lennie pulled at his crotch and tried to read Weldon's face, tried to see what he meant by that.

"Yeah, tells me what to do all the time. Stuff like that."

He must not mean what Lennie thought. "Where's your real daddy?"

"Forget about him. Spends most of his time on that shrimp boat. When he's home, he's usually drunk. For all the good he does, Ma oughta throw him out. Drinks up everything he makes." He shook his head.

"He's a shit...Raymond said that's why he has to work all the time. Somebody's gotta feed the rest of us. Ray spends all his time in that stinkin' hardware store. He's a sucker for the overtime shifts."

Lennie smirked. "I heard somethin' else about Raymond. One of the guys told me he's real big. Is that true? Is he big?"

"Big?"

"Yeah. You know…his thing."

Weldon grinned. "Oh, that. It's big all right—like a damn donkey. Guess we both got that from our daddy."

"Yours is big, too?"

Weldon stood up and stretched his shoulders around. He was still grinning from ear to ear. "That's what they tell me in the locker room."

"How big is it?"

"Well...I guess it's bigger than most of the other guys. I don't know exactly how big. I never measured it."

"You want to measure it?" Lennie asked.

"I wouldn't mind. Only, I don't have a ruler."

"I've got one in my notebook. You want to use it?"

Weldon pulled Lennie up from the grass where he'd been sitting. "I tell you what, let's measure both of 'em. Mine and yours. Okay?"

Lennie felt a tightening in his pants. He looked around. "Right here? Somebody might see us."

Weldon shook his head. "Naw, not here. I know a place down by the bayou. Come on."

"You want to go out there right now?"

"Yeah. Get on your bike and let's go."

Lennie remembered what his mama had always told him. "I have to be home before dark."

"Come on. We've got plenty of time. The place I know about is at that bayou on this side of Lake Boeuf. Get your bike—I'll race you out there."

❖ ❖ ❖

19

Recovery

Must be a dream, Jeremy imagined. Some kind of crazy dream. Why else would he be floating in this white space? Suspended in a vacuum, somehow restrained inside it. When he tried to move, he couldn't raise his left arm. When he looked to see why, sharp pain shot through his head. His arm was tied to a bed, but what the hell was that other stuff? Looked like IV tubing…IV tubing, what the…?

He tried to sit up, but his belly hurt too bad. Ruptured spleen—something like that? Then he discovered he couldn't move his right hand, and he turned to see.... That did it. He knew, then, he was dreaming…he thought it was Barbara holding his hand. Struggling to open his eyes wider, he stretched his eyebrows upward, but pain tore through his head and he struggled to free himself.

"Hold still, Jeremy. You're okay now."

Sounded like Barbara. He did hold still. At least he could hear without causing pain.

"What happened?" His voice cracked. He coughed, and pain sliced through every part of his body. "What the hell is going on? What is this place? Where am I?"

"Hush, Jeremy. Lie still. You're in the staff infirmary."

It was Barbara.

"You've been unconscious. Lie still now. Try to rest."

Slowly, piece by piece, it all began to make sense. He remembered Mrs. LeCompte, remembered trying to keep her from dying. Talking to her husband and the others. The three of them all over him like a swarm of angry hornets. Then, exhausted, he drifted off again.

When he awoke Barbara was still there. Barbara and somebody else…who was that? Looked like Dr. Burton, the Chief of Neurosurgery. Jeremy forced his eyes to focus. It was Dr. Burton. At the foot of the bed, talking to Barbara.

Dr. Burton looked in his direction. "Hello, Jeremy. It's a good time for you to wake up. I need to examine you." He pulled a penlight from his coat pocket and flashed it in and out of Jeremy's eyes. Using a few instruments from the bedside table, he performed a complete neurological exam. Normal, as far as Jeremy could make out. Burton unwrapped a huge blood-stained bandage from Jeremy's head, then poked around on his scalp. That's where the worst pain was—right in the middle of his damn head.

"So far so good," Dr. Burton said. "Everything looks stable. You never had any localizing signs, but you were unconscious almost twelve hours. That's not so good."

"Twelve hours? How bad is it? What about my residency? Will I be able to stay in the program?"

"I believe you will—based upon what I see right now." The neurosurgeon pulled a chair to the side of the bed and sat down to write in a medical record. Jeremy realized it had to be his medical record. He was the patient—that would take some getting used to.

Dr. Burton must have known there'd be empty holes in Jeremy's memory, because he started filling in the blanks. "It's a good thing that lab technologist came along when he did. Looks like he stopped your patient's family before they did too much damage." Dr. Burton looked up from his notes. "Who was your rescuer, anyway? Do you know? Nobody seems to know his name."

Jeremy shook his head. He couldn't remember anything about a lab technologist.

"No matter. Whoever it was, he probably saved you from a much more serious injury."

Jeremy thought about that for a while. "What happened to the people who beat me up?"

"The security police got psychiatry involved. Took 'em a couple of hours to get those three calmed down. Acute situational anxiety, they called it." He looked at Jeremy. "I believe you could bring charges against them if you want to."

"No, I don't want to do that. Normally they're harmless—nice people really. Just a bunch of emotional Cajuns."

"You're right, I guess." Dr. Burton touched Jeremy's arm. "The security folks thought the guy who broke up the fracas was a lab tech because he had one of those blood drawing trays, but they didn't get his name. He disappeared when they took you down to the ER. Your skull x-rays were negative. I sewed up a jagged laceration in your scalp. A lot of bleeding there, but no other open wounds. You did a pretty good job of protecting yourself."

Jeremy smiled. From what he remembered it was a damn poor job.

"We got a CAT scan of your head," Burton said. "It looks okay. The thoracic surgeons tell me you have a couple of broken ribs, but no complications so far. Your head injury is a mild concussion. I expect you to recover fully, but you're going to need at least two weeks of rest."

"Two weeks? Dr. Burton, how can I do that? You know what the schedule's like on the surgery teams."

"It's necessary, Jeremy. I've already spoken to your chief about it. He had the chief resident assign all of your patients to the others for two weeks. Said he'll play it by ear after that. Don't worry about it, it's all arranged."

"Okay." No use to worry anyway, Jeremy decided. There was nothing he could do about it. "Thanks for taking care of everything."

Dr. Burton grinned. "I figured it was the least I could do for a resident injured in the line of duty. We don't give Purple Hearts around here."

Jeremy managed a weak smile. Barbara looked at the two of them and shook her head.

"By the way," Dr. Burton said, "I spoke to your father this morning. He wanted to drive over here right away, but I convinced him to wait a day or two. He wants to take you home to Beaumont, but I can't let you travel before Friday. Don't make any plans until I give you the word."

"All right. Would you mind calling Dad again? Let him know I'm conscious. Tell him not to worry, I'll be fine." He smiled at Barbara. "Maybe I can get Miss Allison to take care of me until Dad gets here."

Barbara winked. "I'll take care of you, all right. You won't do anything unless Dr. Burton says it's okay."

The neurosurgeon gathered up his examining instruments. "I want you to stay in bed until tomorrow, Jeremy. You need rest. That's about all we can do now—lots of rest and time to heal." He turned to Barbara. "Don't worry if he sleeps a lot. That's to be expected for the next day or two."

He did sleep most of the day, awakening for only a few minutes at a time. During one of those times Barbara told him she was leaving to get some sleep herself. Tomorrow was Monday and she was scheduled to work. She pushed his hair off his forehead, then leaned over and kissed him gently.

Nice. He wished.... But he faded into sleep before he could even complete that thought.

The next day came too soon. Jeremy woke up when the infirmary nurse sang out, "Good morning." She breezed into the room and opened the blinds at the window.

Jeremy groaned. Just getting his eyes open was all he could manage, and the bright sunlight was too much. Every part of his body ached—everything he moved hurt so much he wondered if that old cliché were true: like he'd been run over by a freight train.

The nurse checked his vital signs and neurological status. She didn't offer Jeremy any information, but she seemed satisfied. "You wouldn't believe the company you've had. Such a popular guy."

"I hurt too bad to care about that." He did manage a sleepy grin while his sluggish brain tried to catch up with the nurse's remarks. "Who was here? What time is it anyway? Seems early for visitors."

"Early? The day's half gone, it's already past nine." She pulled several loose scraps of paper from her pocket and shuffled through them. "Barbara Allison was here. Now that was early—she's working today." She looked up and grinned. "Barbara didn't want to wake you up, said she'll be back after three. Dr. Burton was here, and the Chief of Surgery—both on their way to the operating room. They'll come by later." She rearranged the pieces of paper and handed several of them to Jeremy. "Four medical students and two residents came to wish you well—here're their names."

The energetic nurse was too full of chatter for Jeremy's aching head. He was glad when she left him alone with a light breakfast. After a couple of bites he fell asleep again.

Then, suddenly, he was awake—wide awake and hungry. His headache was gone and, for the first time, his thinking was clear. Responding to some small sound, some presence, he rolled over and saw a man standing close to his bed. "Guidry. What are you doing here? I didn't hear you come in."

Guidry wore his housekeeping uniform, the gray coveralls, but he didn't seem interested in cleaning the room. He was just standing there with a big grin on his face.

"I'm on my lunch break. Heard you were doing better, but I wanted to see for myself. Looks like them people beat you all to hell, Dr. Becker."

"Thanks for coming by. I'm okay now." What the hell was this all about? He barely knew Guidry. He was not somebody he expected to visit. "Guidry...uh...who told you I was hurt?"

The housekeeper smiled. "It's all around the hospital. Everybody's worried about you, Dr. Becker. The others asked me to find out how you—"

The door burst open and the nurse's honey-coated voice preceded her into the room. "Hello, hello. Lunch time." She positioned Jeremy's lunch tray dead center on the over bed table and started to arrange his bed for eating, then she reacted to Guidry's uniform. Drawing herself up to full height, she glared at Guidry like he'd forgotten who was in charge here. "You'll have to clean the room later. Dr. Becker has to eat his lunch now."

"He's a visitor," Jeremy said. "He's not here to clean he room. Why don't you sit over there, Guidry. Let's talk while I eat."

The nurse shrugged. She stuffed an extra pillow behind Jeremy's back and lifted the warmers from the plates on the lunch tray. "You eat all of this, now. You didn't touch your breakfast." She patted his hand and turned to leave, but not without a disparaging look at Guidry as she headed for the door.

Jeremy was hungry—the food smelled good. He smiled at his visitor and picked up his fork. "Well, Guidry, you really get around the hospital, don't you? How long have you worked here?"

"Fifteen years. Best job I ever had. Nobody in my family ever made it to the city to stay, nobody before me I mean."

That was all Guidry said, then he just sat there. Jeremy figured it would be up to him to keep the conversation going. Between bites of a cheese omelet he said, "Where do you live, anyway? Are you married?"

Guidry laughed. "Lord, no. I ain't married. I live by myself, over by Carrolton and Napoleon Avenue."

Jeremy raised his eyebrows. Dammit, he forgot how bad it hurt to do that. "I guess they call you to take the extra shifts, huh? Because you live alone. What do you do besides work?"

"Not too much. I like to read, and I try to take some night courses at the business college when I can." He grinned. "I'm goin' for manager of the housekeepin' department."

"That's great." Hard to understand a career goal like that, Jeremy thought, but he tried to sound encouraging. "Where does your family live?"

"They used to live in Thibodaux. I grew up down there, came to New Orleans a year or two after I graduated. You ever been to Thibodaux, doc?"

"I think so," Jeremy said. "Wouldn't I drive through Thibodaux on the way to Morgan City? I went down there for a Shrimp Festival a couple of years ago."

Guidry beamed. "Yeah, you probably did go right through Thibodaux if you took Highway 20 out of Vacherie. It's a real nice town."

"I remember it. Clean looking place." Jeremy wasn't at all sure he did remember Thibodaux, but he wanted to keep Guidry talking so he could eat. He really was hungry.

Guidry gazed out of the window. "My family was real poor, Doc. My brother died around the time I was born. It was just the two of us, and I never knew him. My daddy was a shrimper."

"Must be tough trying to get ahead in a small town like that."

Guidry nodded. "I reckon. My daddy never did too much for us, but we made it. It was real hard on Mama. That poor woman spent most of her life running the house and tryin' to make ends meet."

Jeremy shook his head. "Is she still in Thibodaux?"

"Naw…she died a long time ago. Mama deserved a whole lot more'n she ever got. She never had even been...." Gazing out of the sunny window, Guidry drifted off into an absent-minded reverie.

Jeremy felt like an intruder. He knew he needed to change the subject—to bring Guidry back to reality. Talking about his mother must have triggered powerful memories. "Why'd you come to New Orleans, Guidry? How come you started working at Charity?"

Guidry grinned. "You like the old name, too, don't you, Doc? I sure ain't changing it. It's been Charity a mighty long time. Just as soon it stay Charity."

Jeremy chuckled. "I know what you mean. How'd you get started here?"

"A man from Thibodaux got me the job." Guidry glanced at his watch. "Hey, I gotta go. My lunch hour's almost over."

"Okay, Guidry." Jeremy held out his hand. "Thanks for coming by. I enjoyed the visit."

"That's okay. Let me know if I can do anything, hear. Just tell any of the housekeepers you want to see me."

"There is one thing, Guidry. They told me somebody from the lab pulled those people off me the other night. Let me know if you hear anything about who it was. I'd like to thank him."

"Lab? I don't know none a them...." Guidry faded away again. He looked down at the floor and didn't say anything for a long time.

Did his face flush? Jeremy couldn't be certain, but it did look like it. Strange guy.

"Oh, sure...sure," Guidry finally said. "I'll let you know if I hear anything at all about who it was."

"Thanks. Oh, by the way, Guidry, what's your first name?"

"Leonard. Most of 'em call me Lennie."

Jeremy welcomed the chance to doze off after Guidry left. Sleeping so much like that, he lost track of time. When he woke up the nurse was standing by his bed, and he looked up to see what she was doing. He realized, then, it was not the infirmary nurse. It was Barbara, still in uniform.

She smiled and touched his hand. "Hi, sleepy head. I haven't had a chance to tell you how much I enjoyed our evening out. Sorry I slept through your leaving on Saturday morning."

"I left pretty early." He reached for her hand and raised her fingers to his lips. "I tried to be quiet. You were sleeping like a baby."

Barbara laughed, "Oh sure—quite a baby." She ran her fingers through his hair, then drew back when she touched the stitches. She smiled and kissed him on the cheek. "I found your note when I woke up. I got here a little before noon on Sunday. It really blew me away when Joe answered your page. I thought he was making a bad joke when he told me you were unconscious in the infirmary." She straightened the sheet and touched his shoulder. "Never a dull moment with you is there?"

"I guess not…sorry about that."

She finger-combed the front of his unruly hair. "Don't worry about it, Jeremy. You're worth it."

20

Cypress Knees

LENNIE AND WELDON WENT DOWN TO THE BAYOU A LOT AFTER that first day. Three or four days most weeks. After school was out for the summer they went every day. Weldon had to work at the hardware store, but Lennie would always be there waitin' for him when he got off.

Carrizo cane grew thick all around that part of the bayou and made it private. Weldon had chopped a clearing in the middle of a cane patch, like a little room with a crooked hall leading into it. Lennie brought an old trunk from Miss Rena's garage to keep their stuff in and a quilt to put down over the leaves for a soft floor. They always left their clothes in the cane room when they went swimmin', just in case anybody came along. Figured they could hide in the cattails if they had to, and if the meddlers didn't see any clothes layin' around they wouldn't know anybody was there.

It was a good hideout. The bayou widened out right there, and it made a good place to swim. Weldon said his daddy had showed it to him, even took him swimmin' there one day when he was about seven years old. Nobody else knew about it, least ways they never saw any sign of anybody else.

A big cypress tree growin' on one side of the bayou shaded it a little in the middle of the day. Sometimes they made a game out of seeing which one could stand up the longest on top of one of those cypress knees stickin' up in the edge of the water.

That first day, the measuring day, was not supposed to be a contest, though if it had been, Weldon would have won. He was right about being big. But it took more than big to win in the sex games they played. Lennie took the lead. He called the plays, and he was usually the active player.

When Lennie was with Weldon he didn't think much about his past. Not about the stuff with his daddy and not about the way Marshall treated him either. But, as he grew older, he acted like those things had left some ideas in his head. Ideas about how things ought to be between two people. It just seemed natural that he took the upper hand right away with Weldon. Weldon must have liked it that way, because he went along with all of it.

Through the weeks of that first summer, Lennie figured out he could get Weldon to do just about anything he wanted. He used Weldon. Not just the sex, he used him in a lot of other ways, too. Always had Weldon doin' for him, and Weldon acted like he couldn't get enough of it.

They never did tell anybody what they were up to, how much time they spent together or anything. Sometimes Lennie talked Weldon into skipping work at the hardware store. Told him to get his brother, Raymond, to cover up for him so Weldon could come over to Miss Rena's to help with his chores. He knew Weldon would do some of the heavy work for him.

Weldon still wouldn't go inside Miss Rena's house. Wouldn't come over there at all until Lennie figured out a way to slip him in the garden from the alley behind the garage. Nobody in the house could see it wasn't Lennie doing the work out there, and Weldon said he didn't mind. Shoveling and all that would keep him in shape. He told Lennie he liked helping him out, liked the way Lennie teased around while he was working.

One day Lennie was watching Weldon dig up a new part of the garden for a few rows of lettuce Miss Rena wanted. He liked to watch Weldon with his shirt off, shoulder muscles tight. He put down his own hoe and slid his fingers through the sweat on Weldon's back, then headed for the tall bushes at the edge of the garden.

"Got to pee," he said, standing where Weldon couldn't keep from seeing him. When he finished, he slipped his dungarees down to his ankles. Already barefooted, he stepped right out of 'em. Weldon grinned when Lennie started playing with his dick—sorta jerkin' off. "Come on over here, Weldon. Come over here and suck it for me."

Weldon glanced toward the house. "Not here. Let's go down to the bayou."

Lennie cracked a big smile and wriggled his hips a little to make his boner wave around. "Come on. Miss Rena can't come out here. You know that."

"What about the colored man?"

"Don't worry none about Lucifer, he's at the store. You don't have to be scared of him, anyway. He knows I can get him in trouble with Marshall."

"What do you mean? What kinda trouble could an old man like him get into?"

"I found out he's been stealing food, givin' it to his people on the other side of town. No big deal, but I scared him about it." Lennie slipped his shirt over his head and stood there, butt naked in the broad daylight. "Come on, I want you to suck it."

Pants bulging, Weldon stuck his shovel in the ground. He moved Lennie farther back into the bushes and pulled him down to the soft dirt underneath.

It went on like that between them. Even in the winter there were a lot of days warm enough to go down to the hideout, sometimes warm enough to swim in the bayou. On the cold days Weldon would jump in the water if Lennie dared him to do it, then run all around naked to dry off.

They were happy together and, as far as they could tell, nobody knew their secret. The best time of all was that summer before their senior year in school. Weldon was gonna be on the first string and he had to go to football camp for two weeks before school started. By then, he had just about stopped working at the hardware store. He'd figured out how to get Raymond to give him some money, then he'd tell his ma it was his own pay.

Lennie wanted to make something big outa the last day of that summer, so he brought the rest of a chocolate cake from Miss Rena's kitchen and tied some Dr. Peppers in a crab net in the bayou to keep 'em cool. Then he waited for Weldon to get off from the hardware store—it was his last day and he had to be there to pick up his paycheck.

When he got to the bayou Weldon told Lennie his brother, Raymond, knew about their hideout. "He followed me down here the other day."

"Why'd you let him do that, Weldon. I told you we had to keep it a secret."

"I didn't let him do nothin'. I didn't even know he was followin' me. He told me about it later on."

"Sneakin' bastard. What'd he say?" Lennie didn't pay much attention to the answer. He was trying to figure some way to get back at Raymond—to make sure he stayed quiet. Steal some money from the hardware store and blame it on him, something like that.

"He told me he watched us," Weldon said. "Saw us swimmin' and all." He looked down at the ground. "He saw us fuckin' in the cane room."

"Oh shit. What's he gonna do? What did he say?"

"He won't do nothin. I b'lieve he got a kick outa watching us. I begged him not to say anything to Ma or anybody."

"What did you tell him?"

Weldon grinned. "I cried. Carried on about me being his little brother and all. How him and me need to stick together. You'd a been proud of the way I did it. I had to do him a big favor, then finally Raymond said he wouldn't tell a soul."

"You did good, Weldon. Real good." He slipped his arm around Weldon's shoulders. "Let's go swimming."

They took off their clothes and put 'em in the cane room, then ran out naked into the sun. Dodging cypress knees, they frolicked into the water. Weldon won their swimming race to the cattails and back, but it was close. Lennie was right behind him.

After a while, Lennie stood up in knee deep water. "Hey, Weldon, I've got somethin' over here for you if you dive out of that big ol' cypress tree."

"Shoot, you know I can have that thing anyway. I don't have to dive nowhere." He tackled Lennie and they wrestled around in the shallow water.

"Come on, Weldon, dive for me. I dare you."

Weldon let him go and looked up at the big tree. "I bet I could dive off that first limb. If I push off real good I could make it out to the deep water."

"I dare you to do it. Come on, I'll boost you up in the tree."

Weldon grabbed Lennie's shoulders and threw him down in the water. "I don't need no boost. You stay here and watch me."

He scampered up the tree like a monkey up a pole, then eased out on the first limb. "It looks pretty high from up here."

"Come on, you can do it."

"The bark's breakin' off the limb. I can't go out far enough."

"Dive, Weldon. Dive. I dare you."

Weldon grinned down at Lennie, then flew off the limb like a beautiful, naked hawk. His sleek body straight and stiff, he soared through the air. His black hair flew behind like a horse's mane. His head made a loud hollow sound when it hit the cypress knee just under the surface of the brown water. His body crumpled and he disappeared into the bayou. He didn't come up.

21

Doppelgänger

THAT WAS THE ONE ALL RIGHT, BED EIGHT. The ward was dark, but he knew the layout. Bed Eight was the same on all the wards. Right at the end, under the clock. Fifteen beds on every ward. Seven on each side, number eight right in the middle.

The name he had was Jeff Thompson and the clipboard said Bed Eight, but he'd better ask the patient his name anyway. He liked to do that every time, just to be sure.

Sacre! He was young. Looked like...no, couldn't be. What he could see of the man's body looked the same all right, smooth and sleek. But even in the dark ward he could see this one had yellow hair. It made him think about it all the same, bein' so young and all...probably naked under that sheet.

The whole scene made him think about that day he had pulled Weldon naked out of the bayou. He had seen him dive off that limb. He'd known right away he could never make it to the deep water. Weldon must have known better, too. He never would have done it if he hadn't dared him to. Divin' like that, naked as a jay bird.

When he didn't come up after that dive, his brother, Raymond, ran out from his own hidin' place, ran right out in the bayou with his clothes on. By that time Lennie had his arms around Weldon, pullin' him over to the edge. Lennie was naked, too.

"What's wrong with 'im?" Raymond screamed. "Why don't he stand up?"

"What are you doin' here, you bastard? Get the fuck outta my way so I can take care of Weldon. He told me you'd been sneakin' around here, spyin' on us." Lennie pulled Weldon up on the weeds at the edge of the bayou.

"He's out cold," Raymond yelled, shaking his brother's shoulders. "Wake up, Weldon. Do somethin', Lennie. Make him wake up."

Lennie touched Weldon's face. "I don't know what to do. We need some help. Run get somebody to help us, Raymond. Run to the fire station."

Raymond took off. Dripping water from his wet clothes, he ran like the wind, right out through the cane to the edge of town, then on to the fire station.

Four firefighters came back with Raymond. They carried their long board and some kind of satchel down to the water from their ambulance. When they got to the bayou Lennie was kneeling there, right beside the lifeless Weldon. He had put his own clothes back on, and he'd pulled a pair of pants on Weldon.

The firefighters got Weldon strapped on their board and carried him up to the road. He still wouldn't open his eyes or nothing. They put Weldon in the back of the ambulance and pushed Lennie and Raymond in the front seat with the driver. They took off fast and headed for the hospital at high speed, siren wide open.

The nurses told Raymond to go get his mama and bring her to the hospital. Weldon was pretty bad off, they said. When Ray and his mama got back, the doctors had put Weldon in a room and hooked up all their machines. He was lying there like he was asleep, 'cept for all them tubes coming out of him. Lennie was standin' next to the bed, right beside him, touchin' his hand.

Weldon's mama threw a fit. She musta suspected something, 'cause she tore into Lennie like a wet hen. Jerked him away from the bed, pushed him all the way to the door and right on out in the hall. "You stay outa here. Don't you ever come around my boy again. You ain't no better than that sorry old man of yours." Lennie knew Weldon always had been his mama's favorite, she looked after him. She wanted him to study for a priest.

Shoot, Weldon never would of made a priest. He liked what he did with Lennie too much for that. But his ma didn't know that part of it. She never would know it, either…unless that bastard, Raymond, broke his promise.

The doctors said Weldon might live, but he was paralyzed. He wouldn't ever be able to move anything from his neck down. His mama was so sick with grief she couldn't stay with Weldon. She couldn't even come to the hospital very much, but Lennie came. He came to Weldon's room every single day.

He watched all the stuff they had to do to Weldon...it wasn't natural, all them tubes and everything. The breathin' machine was the worst part—breathin' in and out for him all the time like that. They said Weldon would die if he didn't have it, so it kept on huffin' and puffin' at the side of the Weldon's bed like an evil giant or somethin'.

Four weeks later Weldon was no better, and Lennie felt like it wasn't even his friend anymore. Like Weldon was already dead or somethin'. Lennie thought maybe God was punishin' Weldon for what the two of 'em did in their cane room down by the bayou. But Lennie thought he'd been punished enough. He couldn't let his friend stay like that any longer.

He looked at Weldon's face for a long time. So peaceful lookin'. He pulled a comb out of his own pocket and combed Weldon's hair, then leaned down and kissed him on the forehead. While he was close like that, he unhooked the breathin' machine from that tube in Weldon's nose. He stood up then, and stared out of the window, tears runnin' down his face.

A voice came from behind him. "I saw what you did to Weldon."

He jerked upright and spun around toward the voice. "Raymond! What the hell are you doing here? I didn't see you come in."

"Course not, I was in the closet. Ran in there when I heard you comin' in the room 'cause I wanted to see what y'all do when nobody's here. I cracked the door open just wide enough to watch you. I saw you unhook that breathin' machine. You killed my brother, Lennie. I saw you do it."

"I couldn't leave 'im like that—all those machines, him not even knowin' what was goin' on.

"You know Ma told you not to come around here anymore."

"I couldn't stay away from Weldon. You oughta know that. I came to see him every day. I hid in the closet same as you whenever I heard somebody comin'."

"I know you did," Raymond said. "I saw you here a lot—saw you watching what the nurses were doin' and all."

"So you sneaked around, too, and you figured out I spent a lot of time here. So you saw what I did for Weldon. So what? What're you gonna do about it? What're you gonna do, Raymond?"

"I don't know yet," Raymond said. "Weldon might be better off this way."

"That's why I did it, Ray. Don't you know that?"

"Listen to me, Lennie. Don't you ever forget what I saw you do. If you forget it for one minute, I'll tell Ma you killed Weldon. She don't like you anyway, and she'll believe me when I tell her what I saw. Don't you ever forget that."

And neither one of them ever did forget it. Lennie took Weldon's job at the hardware store and tried to be Raymond's friend, but that didn't work out. Raymond drank too much and the sex was no good. Lennie moped around a lot until Marshall Boudreaux told him about a guy he knew over in Golden Meadow—a doctor's son named Dan Hebert, just about Lennie's age. He hitched a ride over there one day to meet Dan, and the two of 'em hung out together for a few months.

Then Lennie left Thibodaux about a year later. Marshall Boudreaux wouldn't let him live at his house in Metairie after Lennie told him he didn't want to go to college. Marshall told him he'd still look after him, but he couldn't live with him and his wife unless he went to school, so he just bummed around New Orleans for a couple of years. Marshall kept on tellin' him things about Dan Hebert, but Lennie didn't see Dan anymore for a while.

When the Health Protection law came in, Lennie had tested HIV-positive. It had been hard to get a job after that. Finally Marshall had put him in touch with some guy he knew who got him a low-paying post in the housekeeping department at Big Charity.

But all of that was a long time ago, and the yellow-haired man in Bed Eight was not Weldon. Him bein' young and all sure made him think about Weldon, but he didn't look a bit like Weldon when he got close enough to see his face in the dark ward. Anyway, he knew what he had to do. He put the lab tray down on the bed and pulled a rubber tourniquet out of his pocket.

The yellow-haired man opened his eyes and looked around in the dark. "What do you want? What are you doing here?"

"Are you Thompson?" Lennie looked at the paper on his tray. "Jeff Thompson?"

"Yes, I'm Thompson. Who are you?" He glanced up at the lighted clock on the wall. "Why are you here in the middle of the night?"

"I'm from the lab. I have to draw some blood." He straightened out Thompson's bare arm and fastened the tourniquet around it just above his elbow.

"Wait a minute. What kind of test is this? I don't think I'm supposed to have any blood drawn at three o'clock in the morning."

What kind of test? Lennie hadn't planned on a question like that, and he didn't know what to say. "I don't know—whatever it says on the slip. I just draw the blood."

"Show me the slip. I want to see what it says. Why in the hell is it set up for the middle of the night?" Thompson reached right in the lab tray and pulled out the only slip in there. "Shine your flashlight on this thing so I can read it."

Lennie didn't like it, but he did what Thompson said. He didn't know what else to do.

"Blood culture," Thompson read. "You guys are crazy. I'm not supposed to have a blood culture."

"Your name's on the slip, ain't it?"

"I don't give a fuck what's on your slip. I'm not having any blood culture." Thompson jerked his arm free and rolled over. "Nurse! Nurse! Help me! Get over here quick!"

Merde! Shit! Lennie was scareder than hell for sure. He had to get out of there in a hurry. He grabbed the lab tray and ran for the hall, somehow ducking around the corner just before the nurse reached Thompson's bed. He kept on running down the dark hall to the nearest stairs, then raced down two floors where he stopped to listen for a minute or two. He heard nothing, no footsteps, nobody chasing him. Relieved, he ambled over to an elevator that would take him to the basement—back to safety in the basement, safe like that day Marshall Boudreaux had held him tight when he was a boy.

❖❖❖

22

Dr. Becker The Elder

Jeremy's father arrived in New Orleans on Wednesday in the early afternoon. At sixty-one he was still a tall, good-looking man who had worked at keeping his body from going stocky. His reddish-blond hair was turning gray, but he had kept the fresh-faced look of a Minnesota farm boy.

Life in a smaller city suited Dr. Becker. After earning his M.D. from Tulane and completing a family practice residency in San Antonio, he had jumped at the opportunity to associate with an older practitioner in the eastern Texas town of Beaumont. When his partner died he inherited the practice, and for nearly thirty years he had nurtured it like an attentive mother hen. The practice had become a part of his life that was difficult to leave, and it took something like Jeremy's head injury to get him to close the office for a few days.

He was HIV-negative and he had anticipated trouble getting into Charity, or whatever it was called those days. He was prepared to plead special circumstances because of Jeremy's injury. A phone call before arriving had set up an security guard escort through the M-E-P to the administrative section, but Dr. Becker feared the worst when he read the neat gold letters on the outer door:

T. Laurence Lockhart, MBA, FACHA
Administrator

Anybody with a name like "T. Laurence" was bound to be a stickler for details, a tedious man to do business with. Especially somebody who put his credentials in gold on the front door. Any remaining hope for a quick agreement vanished when he finally got a look inside Lockhart's office.

The large room was much too sumptuous for Charity Hospital, too much even after they named it Medical Center of Louisiana. The lighting was subdued and the room smelled of furniture polish. Damask drapes over sheer curtains covered the double windows behind Lockhart's desk, itself a regal expanse of gleaming walnut. An Italian library table stood at one side, adjacent to a walnut bookcase, ready for conferences with small groups of his courtiers. A group of antique botanical prints in burl frames with lemon yellow mats hung above the bookcase in a symmetrical arrangement .

Several chairs, all of them tastefully upholstered in fabric earth tones, sat here and there: around the conference table, near Lockhart's desk, and in a conversational grouping alongside a lamp table near the door. The Administrator's own chair, the single exception to fabric upholstery, was an enormous burgundy leather throne.

Lockhart was a tall, thin man with a beak-like nose protruding from a large round face that didn't appear to fit the rest of his body. About forty-three, Dr. Becker guessed. The man's gangly appearance was heightened by limbs that kept moving in a discoordinated way as he flitted in and out of his chair. His constant motion brought to mind a young tree in high wind.

Dr. Becker was right about Lockhart being a stickler. He couldn't reason with the man, could not convince him that Jeremy's injury was sufficient grounds for an exception to the letter of the law about entering the HIV-positive hospital.

"Dr. Becker, you know the Health Protection Act is very specific about these things," Lockhart said. "We are not permitted to allow HIV-negative persons to have access to our patients, certainly not an HIV-negative physician."

"Be reasonable, Lockhart. I won't be involved with any of your hospital's patients except my son, and I won't be treating him. I'm fully aware of the HIV restrictions, but I assure you there is no possibility of virus transfer in either direction as a result of my presence. I'll be happy to sign a release of liability if that'll make you feel better."

Lockhart smoothed the sides of his already neat hair and glanced into a walnut-framed mirror hanging near the desk. "Doctor, you must understand—"

Dr. Becker stood up and leaned over Lockhart's desk. "Listen, I understand your rules very well, but I've never known a rule that didn't have some exceptions. Surely you can do something."

Lockhart waved a silver letter opener like an imperial scepter. "I'm afraid—"

"I don't want you to be afraid, Lockhart. I just want you to hear me. I did not drive all the way from Beaumont to be frustrated by your rules. I intend to be with my son."

"I am sorry, but I cannot permit it. The rules are not mine. I cannot waive them for you."

Dr. Becker stepped away from the desk and straightened the lapels of his navy blue blazer. He removed his glasses and put them in his jacket pocket. "I guess I have to remind you that my son was injured in your hospital. If his surgical career is interrupted by his injuries the hospital could have considerable liability."

Lockhart stopped all movement. At that instant he looked like a flamingo standing motionless on one leg. "That's an outrageous suggestion." His hand perched on the telephone and his beady eyes glinted. "Maybe I'd better ask the hospital attorney to join us."

"I don't believe you need to do that. Think about it...we both know what he'll tell us."

Lockhart wilted. He moved back from the phone and slumped in his chair. For a fleeting moment he seemed ready to be compassionate but, just a quickly, he restored the layer of arrogance he'd worn previously. "Really, Dr. Becker. You've asked me to be reasonable. Give yourself the same advice—your attitude leaves me no choice. No choice at all."

Dr. Becker did not offer an excuse. He knew he had beaten the administrator at his own game.

Lockhart telephoned the governor's office in Baton Rouge. Over-long discussions with a series of aides finally produced an authorization for waiver of the entry requirements. He issued Dr. Becker a specially encoded M-E-P card that would allow him to enter the hospital's buildings for one week.

Half an hour later Dr. Becker walked into Jeremy's room in the infirmary. He was delighted to find Jeremy out of bed and looking well.

Barbara was in the room and, after introducing the two, Jeremy said, "How'd you manage to get in here, Dad? I expected you to call me from your hotel or something."

The older man beamed and showed Jeremy his temporary M-E-P card. "I'm still pretty resourceful when I need to be, but I'm afraid I had to do a number on your Mr. Lockhart." He told them about his run-in with the administrator, exaggerating Lockhart's foot dragging to the point of comedy.

Laughing with the others, Barbara said, "sounds like I've been missing something—I've never met Mr. Lockhart. My chief nurse says he's a real put-off, playing up to the trustees all the time."

"I've known his type before," Dr. Becker said. "Shrewd administrator, but he misses the point of what we medical folks think hospitals are all about."

Jeremy smiled. "Come on, Lockhart's not all that bad."

"He sure gave me a bad time. How long has he been at Charity, anyway?"

"Ummm...maybe three years. That's right, three years. I was an intern when he came. We had an acting administrator for a while after the HIV-positive designation, then the Board of Trustees ended their search and appointed Lockhart."

"What rock did they find him under?" Dr. Becker wondered aloud.

"Leave him alone," Jeremy said. "At least he keeps most of the administrative stuff out of our hair."

❖ ❖ ❖

23

A Shared Mystery

Jeremy and his father spent the next half hour catching up on things in Beaumont—telling Barbara about his mother, his sister, Elaine, and other family things. Finally, Barbara stood and touched Jeremy's shoulder. "It's time for you to go back to bed, Jeremy. Remember what Dr. Burton said—plenty of rest."

Jeremy grinned and gave her a snappy salute, before he climbed back in the bed. Dr. Becker took all that in, but he had already concluded that she and Jeremy had more than a casual work relationship. She was poised and unpretentious, at ease in the company of men, and he liked her instinctively.

Barbara folded the sheet over Jeremy's chest then sat in the easy chair where he'd been. "I hope you don't mind a little shop talk, Dr. Becker. There's something new I need to tell Jeremy about—something with one of my patients."

One of her patients, Dr. Becker thought. Strange choice of words for a nurse—very different from his own world of private practice.

Barbara pulled the chair a little closer to the bed. "We had another unexpected death on my ward this morning, Jere. The patient was recovering from a heart attack, just about ready to be discharged, a lot like the others." She looked at Dr. Becker. "He suddenly turned up with high fever, and a few hours later he was dead. The staff did everything possible, but nothing made a bit of difference."

Dr. Becker was caught off guard by Barbara's story. He was a little uncomfortable hearing such details about someone else's patient from a nurse, but he decided to go along with it. "Did the medical staff suggest a reason for the man's sudden turn for the worse?"

"No, sir. No one on the staff could explain his death, but they are going to do an autopsy." She shrugged. "At first we thought it was another infarct, but his EKG was unchanged and he had no chest pain."

Puzzled, uncertain of what they expected him to say, Dr. Becker looked at his son for a clue. Jeremy said, "We've had several deaths under similar circumstances in the past couple of weeks, Dad."

So that was it. He knew Jeremy well enough to realize his tangential approach to the discussion meant he was worried about something. "Surely there's a reasonable explanation for the deaths, Jeremy. What did your staff say about them?"

"I don't think anybody on the staff has considered all of the cases together," Jeremy said. "Taken alone, each one of the deaths could've been some complication of whatever brought 'em to the hospital in the first place." He glanced at Barbara. "The two of us thought about toxic shock, septic thrombophlebitis, pulmonary embolism—things like that."

Dr. Becker removed his blazer and hung it over the back of his chair. "It does sound unusual. Tell me a little more about the cases. Were they all on the same ward? How many deaths have you had, anyway?"

"Five," Jeremy said. "No, six counting the new one Barbara just told us about. They were on several different wards, some medical, some surgical. My own patient was one of them—the woman whose family beat me up." He glanced at the clock on the his bedside table. "Joe should be here soon—you remember Joe Monteleone, my roommate. We believe one of his patients was the first."

"What about AIDS?" Dr. Becker asked. "All of your patients are HIV-positive—maybe the deaths were caused by AIDS."

Jeremy shook his head. "I don't think so. Yes, they're all positive, but we check out the immune system on every patient at the time of admission. I know the surgical deaths had early stage HIV disease. None of them was even close to AIDS." He looked at Barbara. "We could probably find out about the others, couldn't we?"

Barbara nodded. "They all looked early stage to me, but we could review their charts if you want to confirm it."

A short while later, Joe arrived, carrying hangers with a jacket and a couple of shirts. After greeting Dr. Becker he flipped the jacket open to show Jeremy the trousers and tie underneath, then he hung the clothes in the locker beside the bathroom door.

Jeremy said, "Thanks for bringing my things, Joe. We were just telling Dad about the unexplained deaths we've been seeing. Tell him about your Mr. Gilmore."

"Okay, I will. But there's something new I want to tell you first."

"Shoot."

"You remember Jeff Thompson, don't you? That grad student with the suntan and appendicitis?"

Jeremy smiled. "I do remember Jeff. How's he doing?"

"He's fine, but he told us a strange story when we saw him on rounds a little while ago."

"What do you mean, strange?"

"Well...your team told him he should stay in town for a couple of weeks, so he volunteered for one of the HIV protocols. He found out he could transfer to the regional center in Boston for outpatient follow-up."

"Good," Jeremy said. "I hope they put him on that new protocol."

"Whatever," Joe said. He brought a straight chair from the corner of the room and sat down near the bed. "Jeff asked us if we'd ordered any lab studies that needed blood drawn in the middle of the night. No one had, of course." He glanced at Dr. Becker. "He's practically ready to leave the hospital."

"What about the screening tests for the HIV protocol?" Barbara asked. "The residents wouldn't have to order those—the HIV lab does them automatically."

"You're right, but they never draw blood late at night." He grinned. "Those guys are all on Civil Service and they don't work after hours."

"So what happened, Joe?" Jeremy asked. "Quit dragging it out—you're not writing a novel here."

Joe looked slowly around the group. "Well…Jeff told us some guy woke him up at three o'clock this morning—a man wearing hospital clothes. He said it was time for some lab tests and he put a rubber tourniquet on Jeff's arm. The guy had a regular hospital lab tray with syringes and blood tubes and all."

Joe stood and walked to the foot of the bed. "Your team has kept Jeff pretty well informed about hospital routines, Jeremy. He suspected something was wrong, drawing blood in the middle of the night, so he asked the technologist what kind of test the blood was for. Jeff said he got an evasive answer, so he pulled his arm away from the guy. He saw the lab request for a blood culture with his name on it, but he knew which tests were part of the protocol he'd signed up for. He knew blood culture was not one of 'em."

Joe winked at Barbara and sat on the arm of her chair. "Well, Jeff started yellin' in the dark ward, screamin' for the nurse. All the other patients woke up and they started yellin' at Jeff. They must've thought he was still half asleep or somethin'."

Dr. Becker grinned at the image of chaos Joe was building.

Laughing, Jeremy pulled his elbow against his sore ribs. "Ow! Stop it, Joe. That hurts."

"It's not supposed to be a joke. Jeff was really frightened. In the confusion, the lab tech grabbed his tray and took off. Jeff said the man disappeared before anybody got the lights on."

Barbara slid her hand around Joe's arm. "Did you believe Jeff? Maybe he was just trying to be funny."

"The ward nurse didn't believe him. She tried to calm him down—told him he must have had a nightmare. Jeff went along with it, just to get the ward settled." Joe reached into the pocket of his hospital coat and held up a rubber tourniquet. "But if it was a nightmare, what about this thing? The lab tech left it on Jeff's arm when he ran away."

"Damn," Jeremy said. "It's not a joke, is it? Did you report it to anybody?"

"No. I thought about going to the administrator, but Jeff asked me not to. He thought it was just some lab SNAFU, and he's convinced he can take care of anything else that comes up."

"Did Jeff know who the lab tech was?" Jeremy asked.

"No. Said he'd never seen the guy, but he was wearing a hospital coat. Dark hair, Cajun accent. And he had some kind of ID badge on his coat."

"That's no help," Barbara said. "Sounds like about half of the men who work at Charity."

Dr. Becker sat quietly for several minutes, mentally processing the things he'd heard. Finally, he stood and paced around the room, now darkening in the fading evening light. He stopped at the foot of his son's bed. "Jeremy, I was already concerned about security in a hospital that would allow you to be beaten by a patient's family." He looked slowly from one of them to the other. "Then you told me about patients dying unexpectedly, now Joe's story makes it even worse. I don't know what's going on here, but I don't like the sound of it."

Joe and Barbara glanced at each other, then at Jeremy. None of them spoke.

"Who knows about all of this?" Dr. Becker asked. "You said the surgery staff hasn't considered all of the deaths as a group. Has anyone looked into them? It's beginning to sound like some kind of weird epidemic."

Jeremy raised his eyebrows to Joe and Barbara, then looked at his father and shrugged. "To the best of my knowledge there's no plan for any kind of official investigation. Barbara and Joe know my feelings—I don't like it either. I told Barbara I wanted to talk to you about it. I wanted to see what you thought before I took it any further."

Dr. Becker started pacing again. "Okay. Now you've got me involved, so I'll tell you what I think. Somebody should be looking into the whole thing. Since they're not, we need to talk about what we can do." He stopped and looked at Jeremy. "I want to get some hospital official involved in this. Somebody needs to know about it—it could be dangerous."

"Whoa, Dad. You're moving too fast. Maybe it's nothing but coincidence."

"How do you explain the similarity in the cases?"

"I admit they sound similar, but we haven't really checked out the details. I think we ought to review the records—see what we can find there. I hate to make it a federal case before we're even sure there's a problem."

"I don't know," Joe said. "If there is danger, like your father says...."

Barbara took Jeremy's hand. "I agree with your father. We need to be careful."

Dr. Becker said, "The point is, somebody other than the three of you needs to look at the cases you've told me about. If my fears are correct, I'd rather somebody else do the looking."

Jeremy scratched his three-day stubble of beard. "Okay, I guess I'm outnumbered."

Dr. Becker said, "I suggest we keep all of this to ourselves for the rest of the night. I'll see the administrator in the morning. Maybe I can get him to set up an investigation."

"There is one more thing," Jeremy said. "I'd forgotten all about it until I heard Joe's story about the three-AM technologist." He looked at his father. "Some technologist drew blood from Mrs. LeCompte an hour or two before she went bad. Some lab tech drew a blood culture no one had ordered."

"Mrs. LeCompte?" Dr. Becker asked. "Who's Mrs. LeCompte?"

"My patient who died."

"That woman whose family attacked you?"

Jeremy nodded.

"Jesus. I knew there was danger."

"Wait a minute—I'm sure those people didn't have anything to do with the rest of it."

"We can't be sure about anything," Dr. Becker said. "Not yet."

Joe got up and moved to the side of the bed. "Do you realize what you just said, Jeremy. It's the same as my patient—same as Mr. Gilmore. A technologist drew blood from both of 'em just before they died."

"I know." Jeremy looked at Barbara. "Remember what you told me last week about those first deaths on your ward? We talked about it at dinner—something about blood work before they died. Do you remember who drew the blood? Did you tell me who it was?"

"I don't know whether I told you, but I'm sure it was a technologist." She hesitated. "Yes, I am sure—the night nurse said the patients were fine when the lab tech came by to draw blood."

"Damn, Jeremy, you were right," Joe said. "I thought you were crazy, but you were right all along."

Dr. Becker was baffled. "Will you two please tell me what you're talking about. What's so unusual about lab techs drawing blood?"

They reminded him of the hospital's shortage of lab technologists and how rare it was for a tech to be available to draw blood on the wards.

Dr. Becker smiled. "Charity was the same thirty years ago. The budget planners always thought they didn't need lab techs for blood drawing—they told us it was good practice for the students and interns."

"Nothing's changed," Jeremy said. "That's why I thought something odd was going on when all the patients seemed to be doing well until they had blood drawn by a lab tech. After that, they got in trouble in a hurry. They all died a few hours later."

"Jeremy tried to tell our staff about that at the death conference last week," Joe said, "but nobody would listen to him. I'm sorry I didn't help you get it across, Jeremy. I just couldn't see the connection at that time."

"Don't worry about it. The Chief embarrassed me that day—the way he brushed the whole thing off like I was paranoid about blood drawing and needle sticks."

"The Chief also told you he'd check with the lab about technologists being in the ICU before Mr. Gilmore died. Have you heard anything more about that?"

"No, not yet." Jeremy grinned. "It hasn't been a very good week for me, remember?"

"Who was at that conference?" Dr. Becker asked. "Who heard you talking about your suspicions?"

"The whole surgery staff was there," Jeremy said. "House staff, too. And students—the amphitheater was full."

"Who else knows you're worried about the technologists?"

"Nobody. That conference is the only place I've talked about it before tonight."

"Good. I don't mind telling you I'm more than a little concerned about some of the things you've been telling me. Each one of you has been involved in some way with patients' deaths that are too similar to be happenstance. The family of one of them attacked Jeremy. Now this business about lab technologists...I don't like it. Something's wrong. Whatever it is, it could be dangerous. The three of you might be in danger."

"Don't go overboard, Dad. How could we be in danger? You've been reading too many mysteries."

"I won't go overboard—but we are going to get to the bottom of this. I'll see Lockhart first thing in the morning. If he won't order an investigation we'll find some other way to do it."

❖❖❖

24

Fathers and Sons

Back at his hotel, Dr. Becker slept fitfully. Never more than half-asleep, he waffled between thinking about all the things Jeremy and his friends had told him and dreaming about them. Something about the whole thing never did ring true, no matter how objective he tried to be.

Several times he jerked awake in panic from a dream in which he watched, mute and unable to move, while a hideously ugly old woman wearing a shining white uniform circled a hospital bed in the center of a darkened room. In the dream, Jeremy was asleep in the bed and Dr. Becker was unable to warn him that the circling woman had a huge syringe and needle in her hand.

The old crone clenched her empty hand into a fist which she shook at Jeremy in cadence with mumbled phrases of a dirge-like mantra that thundered out of her throat. Each circle brought her closer and closer to the bed until finally she towered over Jeremy's inert body, her grotesque needle poised to puncture his arm. Then, suddenly, the form of the needle changed. It became a slender phallus and laughter erupted from it just as Dr. Becker awoke.

By early dawn he was exhausted, so he gave up the bed in favor of a long hot shower followed by room-service breakfast with the morning paper. Leaving the hotel, he opted for a slow walk to the foot of Canal Street where he wandered into a river boat terminal and bought a plastic cup of bad tasting coffee. He walked along the wharf, searching for order among the chaotic swirls of muddy water at the river's edge. Finally, he took a taxi to the hospital and went directly to the administrator's office.

Lockhart's receptionist was not eager to bend the rules for him—she must have heard about the trouble he'd caused the day before. "Mr. Lockhart and the staff are in their morning report, Dr. Becker. Why don't you come back in about half an hour? I'll ask him then if he can see you."

"I'll wait. I think he'll see me." He turned toward Lockhart's office door. "Come to think of it, the staff might like to hear what I have to say. Maybe I could join them instead of waiting."

The receptionist jumped up and moved between him and the door. "Please, Dr. Becker, just have a seat over there. I'll get you in as soon as I can. This is a very busy time of day." She looked at him and smiled for the first time. "Would you like a cup of coffee?"

"Yes, coffee would be nice. Sweetener, please. No cream." He planned to barge into the office when she left the area, but that opportunity never arose. The receptionist kept a carafe of coffee in a cupboard behind her desk, and she brought him a steaming cup without once letting him out of her sight.

Sooner than he expected the office door opened, and several men in business suits walked out, followed by two nurses in white uniforms. The receptionist darted inside before Lockhart appeared. A few minutes later the two of them emerged, deep in conversation but glancing toward Dr. Becker.

The lanky administrator was dressed like a dandy. His dark gray suit had a European cut, and he wore a red and gray paisley tie with a matching handkerchief arranged like bright plumage in his jacket pocket so that four points of exactly the same height were visible. He strode toward the waiting area, bouncing more than walking, extending his hand as he approached. He acted friendly enough, but his voice had a patronizing tone. "Good morning, Dr. Becker. Miss Faget tells me you're upset about something. What's the matter, didn't your entry card work properly?"

"She's right about being upset." Dr. Becker glared directly at the administrator. "But it's not about anything as mundane as an M-E-P card."

Lockhart stopped and drew back, his head cocked to one side.

Dr. Becker took his time returning the magazine he'd been leafing through to its neat row on the coffee table—let Lockhart wonder for a while. "I've learned of some things that I think you should know about, Mr. Lockhart. You've had a series of unusual events in your hospital. Events that I believe may involve foul play."

"What on earth are you talking about?"

Dr. Becker stood up. "Let's go in your office? I want to talk about some things that I'd rather not discuss in the waiting room."

"Of course." Lockhart looked at his wrist watch as he led the way into the spacious room. "But you'll have to be quick. I can only give you a few minutes." He paused and glanced at Dr. Becker with a smug look. "I'm expected at the mayor's office for a meeting of civic leaders."

Dr. Becker decided Lockhart was the wrong way to reach senior management. Disgusted with the supercilious man and his exaggerated view of his own importance, the doctor stopped just inside the door. "The things I have to tell you will require more than a few minutes, Lockhart. Since you're in such a rush, I'll get the information to you in some other way." He turned to leave. "Meanwhile, perhaps you'd like to tell the mayor your hospital is having an epidemic of unexplained deaths. An epidemic that may threaten the lives of some of your staff."

Lockhart flushed. "What are you talking about? Have the house staff been twisting your imagination with their tall tales?"

"Tall tales? I wouldn't call dead patients a tall tale. And what about visitors who are allowed to beat up the house staff?"

"Really, Dr. Becker. Aren't you getting carried away? We regret your son's injury, but, remember, the residents are young and impressionable. We know they are overworked—they tend to overreact to everyday events."

"I don't believe the families of your dead patients would consider my concerns an overreaction." He hoped the bluff would get Lockhart's attention.

"Oh? You're in touch with the families? Maybe we can talk later in the day." Lockhart began his bouncy walk toward the door. "Let's ask Miss Faget what time...."

"Don't bother. I'll send you a report." Dr. Becker turned and left the office, glad to be out of that place. He had never been able to deal patiently with people whom he viewed as incompetents in positions of authority. This medical center needed a human being in the administrative office, not an unfeeling bureaucrat. He was more determined than ever to get to the bottom of the strange happenings, no matter what it took.

He needed time to settle down, so he chose the stairs to the infirmary rather than the elevator. Opening the door to Jeremy's room, he was startled to find the bed empty. Jeremy was nowhere in sight. Already upset, Dr. Becker was convinced his worst fears had come true—the evil dream had foretold real events.

The bed was bare, sheets removed like the disinfecting routine when a patient dies. Unable to find the call button, he was on the brink of running to the nurses' station when he remembered the adjoining bathroom. He jerked the door open and a cloud of steam rolled out. "Jeremy!" he called.

No answer.

He ran to the shower door and threw it open. His surprised, naked and soaking wet son jumped back from the door, bumping against the tiled wall. "Dad! Don't do that! I didn't hear you come in. I'm trying to wash the blood out of my hair."

"I'm sorry, Son." He shook his head and closed the shower door. "Finish your shower." Damn, maybe Lockhart was right. Maybe he was letting his imagination run wild. Maybe he had been reading too many mysteries. Still....

Hair wet and tousled, Jeremy walked into the room looking like a little boy, wearing only a towel wrapped around his slim body. "Morning, Dad. How's your hotel? Did you sleep okay?"

"I was restless—spent most of the night thinking about the things you guys told me last night."

"I didn't mean to upset you." Jeremy stepped into a pair of briefs, then carefully toweled his hair and combed it with his fingertips. "I'm sorry about yelling at you in there. When you opened the shower door I thought it was the housekeeper. They were supposed to change the bed while I was in the shower."

"Don't apologize, I should have knocked. How are you feeling this morning?"

"Better after the shower. I was getting' pretty grungy."

"I saw Lockhart earlier," Dr. Becker said. "I tried to convince that man he may have a problem, but he basically told me I'm crazy." He shook his head. "He's the crazy one—acts like God's gift to hospitals."

Jeremy pulled on the trousers Joe had brought. "Don't let Lockhart get to you—you know that's what he wants. It makes him feel important. When are you going to learn, Dad? There's no way you can change guys like that. Just blow it off."

"Easy to say." He looked at Jeremy. Was his son suddenly wise enough to teach his father about life? "Why are you getting dressed? You said Dr. Burton doesn't want you to leave until tomorrow. There's no way I'm taking you out of here against his advice."

"Relax, Dad. We're not leaving." He nudged his father into the easy chair. "We're goin' to have lunch in the staff dining room, then we've got an appointment for a tour of the HIV research lab. My chief arranged it last week. It's all set—I talked to him this morning about getting a clearance for you."

"You telephoned the Professor of Surgery for a trivial thing like that?" Dr. Becker asked. Times really had changed since he was at Tulane.

"No, no. I didn't call him. He came by here early this morning. We had a long talk—he sends you his best."

"That's nice. Maybe I should talk to him about your patients' deaths. I'm not getting anywhere with Lockhart."

"No, don't do that. Don't get the Chief involved. I don't want him to think I'm a whiny little kid—I got a licking, now my daddy wants to beat up somebody."

"Don't you think he needs to know about the similarity in those death cases? The things we talked about?"

"I told him about all of that this morning."

"Oh? Come on, Jeremy—you told me I was moving too fast.... What did your Chief say?"

"He's gonna look at the autopsy reports on all of them, then get together with the Chief of Medicine."

"Jeremy, that'll take weeks. You know the final autopsy reports won't be available for—"

"I don't want to tell the Chief how to check it out, Dad. He already thinks I'm overreacting."

"Overreacting about the lab technologists?"

Jeremy nodded. "He told me he found out the lab had a couple of extra techs on duty the night Joe's patient got in trouble. One of them remembers drawing blood in the ICU two or three times during that night."

"That's it, then?"

"The Chief thinks so." Jeremy put on his shirt and buttoned the cuffs. "But he did agree to check the autopsy reports—he'll look for any similar findings."

Dr. Becker shook his head. Was he really such a country bumpkin that he saw problems in the big city hospital where none existed? He didn't think so. "What about this research tour, Jeremy? Are you up to it? How long will it take? You know Burton wants you to rest."

"It's no problem—I feel great. Dr. Burton knows about the tour. The Chief's pretty excited about some of the stuff the lab is doing. He wants us to get our patients to volunteer for testing a new treatment protocol, so I thought I should learn a little more about it." He slugged his father's arm playfully. "Anyway, you know how I feel about new treatments. When something promising comes along I want to be first in line."

Dr. Becker smiled, but said nothing. He and Jeremy had agreed to quit arguing about the wisdom of Jeremy's decision to go through the long years of surgery training after he became HIV positive. He had admired Jeremy's ambition, had even been proud of it, but the father in him had wanted to take his son home, hold him close and protect him. He had finally realized Jeremy would take the residency with or without his blessings, so he decided to support his decision rather than continuing to fuss about it.

Pulling a tie under his shirt collar, Jeremy walked to the bathroom mirror. "I hope you don't mind going to the HIV lab with me. Between their tight security and my work schedule, it took a little planning to set up a tour—I'd sure hate to miss it."

"What do you mean, mind? I'm looking forward to it. I just don't want you to wear yourself out. I've got a healthy respect for head injuries."

"Come on, Dad. I love you for caring, but don't be a worry wart." Jeremy adjusted the four-in-hand knot in his tie. "I'm a big boy now."

"Okay, let's go."

Jeremy picked up a comb and ran it through his thick hair. "Ow! Goddammit—forgot about the sutures. Christ, I'm bleeding. Look at this thing, Dad. See what I did to it."

Dr. Becker separated Jeremy's hair and blotted the scalp wound with a towel. "It's okay. Looks like you snagged one of the sutures. A little pressure should stop the bleeding." A couple of minutes later he lifted the towel. The wound was dry—no further bleeding. He tossed the towel in the sink and swatted Jeremy on the butt. "Ready to go now, big boy?"

"Not until you scrub your hands." Jeremy picked up the towel and put it in the contaminated linen hamper. "Don't forget, my blood can be infectious."

He was a country bumpkin. He put his hands on Jeremy's shoulders. "How do you do it, Son? How do you keep going?"

Jeremy shrugged. "You get used to it. It never gets any easier, but you do get used to it. Now wash your hands while I put on my shoes. Let's get out of here."

25

HIV LAB

SHORTLY BEFORE ONE O'CLOCK JEREMY AND HIS FATHER WALKED through the rear door of the medical center then across the street to the HIV Research Facility. Major renovation had changed the former VA Hospital into a twelve story building that looked more like a garrison than a laboratory. A steel and thick glass guard booth was part of the barrier that blocked access to the heavy looking steel doors that had replaced the traditional entrance. A tight row of vertical steel bars on one side of the guard booth and a pair of flanking concrete buttresses completed the new facade. Just as the two walked up to the booth the amplified voice of a uniformed man seated behind thick glass stopped them. "I need to see your HIV cards, please."

Jeremy inserted his card into a slot on the small counter in front of the booth and smiled at his father when the card popped up inside like a metro ticket. The guard examined the card, glancing back and forth between it and Jeremy's face. He swiped it through a magnetic reader. Moments later the Darth Vader voice of a computer rang out, ***"**Jeremy * D * Becker.**Confirm right thumb print on the lighted screen.**"***

A blue glow appeared on a small screen embedded in the counter. The guard pointed to the screen, and Jeremy pressed his thumb against it. Green light flashed momentarily inside the machine, and the computer spoke again. ***"** Identity confirmed.**Visitor authorized.**Proceed when directed.**"***

The guard repeated the routine with Dr. Becker's card, but the machine responded differently. After reading his thumb print it announced, ***"** Identity confirmed.** LIMITED ENTRY***

ONLY.**" A loud buzzer sounded and a red light flashed angrily on the guard's console.

The guard turned off the warning signals and ran his finger down a list of names on a clipboard. "Dr. Becker, you are cleared for the briefing room only—you won't be allowed to take the full tour of the lab itself."

Jeremy bristled. "What do you mean, won't be allowed? The taxpayers built this place. Why can't he go in? The Professor of Surgery set it up this morning."

The guard shrugged and shook his head. "It's for his own protection. They'll explain it to him after the briefing."

"What do you think, Dad? We don't have to do this."

"Calm down," Dr. Becker said. "Let's go ahead—I know it's important to you. I'll talk to somebody inside."

The guard smiled, more a smirk than a friendly smile, then he turned a key sticking out of his console. The vertical bars beside his booth disappeared into the concrete floor and the building's steel doors slid open. The guard waved them past his station.

Jeremy hesitated, then leaned toward the guard. "Listen, I'm afraid I didn't get very good directions. Can you tell me where to go once we're inside?"

"We don't give information here," the guard said. "Ask the attendant at the desk in the lobby."

Jeremy flushed, but it was nearly time for the briefing, so he squelched the urge to protest and headed for the open door instead. "Bastard," he muttered. "Just like the rest of 'em—won't budge half an inch past his job description."

Dr. Becker laughed. "I can't believe you said that. All those years, I thought you weren't paying attention. Remember what I taught you—don't let 'em grind you down."

Once in the lobby, Jeremy spotted a pleasant looking middle-aged woman at the information desk and headed in her direction. "Can you tell us where to go for the laboratory tour?"

Smiling brightly like she was pleased to be asked, the woman handed him a sheet of paper with printed directions to the Public Briefing Room. "It's right down that corridor toward the rear of the building."

All right, Jeremy thought. Why were volunteers always more helpful than paid employees in bureaucratic institutions?

The heavy doors to the briefing room opened easily, but the room's appearance stopped them in their tracks. Low level indirect lighting gave the whole place a bland, monochromatic look. Everything was beige and soft—rows of plush seats, thick carpeting everywhere, even on the low divider separating the front seats from a speaking platform.

They selected front row center and discovered the seats were like cushioned lounge chairs. The high wall behind the platform was a giant projection screen that curved imperceptibly into the walls on either side of the room. The moment they sat, quiet music from hidden speakers filled the room and the entire projection wall began to glow with soft blue light.

A small door in the carpeted divider slid open directly in front of each seat, exposing a lighted compartment containing a notebook and a pen, both imprinted with the lab's logo. Inside the leather notebook Jeremy found a tightly printed press release on the Regional Lab's letterhead. He nudged his father, who retrieved his own copy, and they both leaned toward the lights to read:

For Release First Week of October.
HIV RESEARCH PRODUCES NEW VIRUS, NOBEL NOMINATION

The Central Regional HIV Research Facility at New Orleans has produced a new strain of the HIV retrovirus that multiplies and mutates a thousand times more rapidly than the standard virus. Officially designated HIV, NOLA strain as a tribute to its city of origin, N.O. LA, the new virus was an accidental discovery that offers real hope of a Nobel prize for the facility's Virology Department.

Retroviruses, including the NOLA strain, are unique among infectious agents. They invade certain cells of the body and make themselves a part of the genetic structure within those cells. At varying time intervals the cells literally explode, releasing large numbers of new virus particles, each of them an exact genetic copy of the virus that invaded the cell. The HIV retrovirus invades cells that are vital to the body's immune system, the T-helper cells. When those cells are destroyed AIDS victims lose their ability to resist diseases that would be trivial to a healthy immune system.

Mutation, which occurs at unprecedented speed in the NOLA strain, is a sudden change in some inheritable characteristic of an organism caused by an alteration of its genetic material. In the HIV, the genetic changes of mutation dramatically influence its response to treatment.

Most drugs used to treat AIDS latch onto the virus's cell membrane or otherwise work themselves into a critical spot in the virus's biochemistry, like a molecular key that fits precisely into a

virus lock. Once in place, the drug alters some vital function of the virus in ways that weaken it or destroy it. But, through mutation, the virus fights back. It changes its biochemistry at the genetic level so that the key no longer fits the lock—the virus becomes resistant to the drug.

The NOLA strain resulted from a treatment trial in the laboratory that did not produce the expected result. Instead, the experimental drug under study seemed to stimulate vastly more rapid mutation. Facility virologists say the drug actually destroyed slower mutating strains and allowed the evolution that isolated and purified the rapid growers. Our researchers determined the laboratory trial had modified the virus genome in a way that accelerated all of its biologic processes without producing any other changes.

The genome is the aggregate of an organism's genes, a cluster of protein building blocks that acts like a control center for all its biologic functions. The New Orleans facility's Genetic Engineering Department has led its peers in mapping the entire genome of the HIV and several related viruses.

Other than its turbo-charged life cycle, the HIV, NOLA strain reacts normally in every way. Its unique life in the fast lane is precisely the reason for NOLA's value. Testing new drugs against NOLA reveals *in vitro* effectiveness, or lack of it, in days instead of months. It tells researchers much more quickly whether they are on the trail of a promising new treatment, or on another wild goose chase.

The potential of HIV, NOLA strain for dramatically shortening the time required to define a safe and lasting cure for AIDS has attracted worldwide scientific interest. It has earned the nomination of NOLA's discoverers for a Nobel prize.

The Nobel Committee, meeting in Oslo, Norway, is expected to announce this year's....

The room lighting dimmed further. Jeremy glanced at his father then put away the press release. Projected images appeared on the screen, faint at first, then brighter. The changing scene depicted medical scourges of centuries past: bubonic plague, cholera, smallpox. Ominous sounding music flooded the room as the scene rolled through time to the twentieth century and depicted syphilis, tuberculosis, polio. The music became triumphant and the lab's motto, ***Knowledge Conquers Adversity***, grew from a central pinpoint to fill the entire screen.

"Can you believe this place?" Jeremy asked. "Can you imagine what they paid for all this high tech stuff?"

Dr. Becker raised his eyebrows and nodded.

The music faded as a carefully modulated voice-over said, "Welcome to the Central Regional HIV Research Facility. This laboratory is one of three in the United States which is dedicated to the single goal of conquering the Human Immunodeficiency Virus, an essential first step in overcoming the group of lethal disorders which we refer to as AIDS, Acquired Immune Deficiency Syndrome." The screen showed production credits over a series of still shots of the HIV Laboratory.

"This whole thing must be automated," Jeremy said. "We're the only people here."

Dr. Becker motioned for Jeremy to stay quiet.

"...is made possible by the concern and dedication of the President of the United States..." Soft undertones of "Hail to the Chief" accompanied cinematography of the White House and the President. "...and of the Congress." The film faded to Capitol Hill and showed leaders of the Congress at work in their chambers. "The wisdom of those officials has provided funding for three regional research institutes. Two billion dollars per year has been appropriated for operation of the three facilities." The camera panned to the research units in Massachusetts and California, then back to New Orleans.

Jeremy moved slightly to cross his legs, and the shape of his seat changed to accommodate his new position. "Did you feel that?" he whispered. "Move around and see what happens to your chair—it hugs your butt. No wonder we don't have a cure yet. This place is a two billion dollar a year Hollywood production for the politicians. It's a propaganda mill."

"Be quiet, Jeremy. I want to hear the rest of it."

"...facility's role in this national battle to conquer the greatest adversity of our time is carried out with the oversight of a Regional Board of Directors, men and women who are recognized leaders in their regions. The Board of Directors for the New Orleans facility is composed of seven outstanding citizens...."

Portraits of each Director appeared on the screen, followed by motion picture clips of each of them in their everyday lives. The biographical sketches continued, "Marshall Boudreaux, prominent New Orleans businessman and entrepreneur, is an ardent supporter of community interests, and he is known for his generous philanthropy. Mr. Boudreaux served as Rex, King of Carnival in...." Pictures of Mardi Gras crowds and a gala ball rolled across the screen. "...other Directors include the Board of Trustees of the former New Orleans Charity Hospital, now called Medical Center of Louisiana at New Orleans."

The audiovisual briefing continued with medical information about the HIV and AIDS. "...in the African green monkey, native to central Africa." A colony of primates was shown in their jungle habitat. "...to the United States during the late 1970s, most likely through the Caribbean nation of Haiti...." Most of that was old news to Jeremy, but the slick presentation held his attention.

A changing collage of moving scenes and harsh headlines kept pace with the continuing narration. "...perceived by many as a 'gay disease.' ...male homosexuals and intravenous drug users.... Many objected to spending large amounts of money...'subsidized sodomy.' By the late eighties...increasingly prevalent in children and heterosexual men, then women. More recently, the epidemic spread of HIV disease among young people alarmed...."

Soft music floated beneath the narrator's dulcet tones. "...the universal nature of the growing threat led to widespread fear of a lethal contagious disease for which the world's health care systems could find no cure, no vaccine. ...conservative groups reversed their positions and joined the battle to defeat a common enemy. Those initiatives led to the Health Protection Act of 1989 which created this Regional Research Facility."

Finally, the music faded and the lights came up. A previously invisible door at one side of the platform opened silently and a tall, slender man emerged. Wearing a white laboratory coat over his shirt and tie, he was clean cut and handsome. His horn-rimmed glasses and a thick shock of light brown hair set off his youthful appearance. Thirty-five or so, Jeremy guessed. Just as the man reached the center of the platform a single spotlight focused on him.

"Good afternoon, Dr. Becker...both of you. My name is Daniel Hebert." He grinned. "I usually work in the Virology Department, but it's my day to be your tour guide. I hope you enjoyed our canned briefing."

When Hebert moved toward them with his hand outstretched, the Beckers stood up, and the lighted compartments in front of their seats closed instantly. Hebert's spotlight was replaced by normal room lighting. "Those damn seats are too much," Jeremy said. "Have you ever electrocuted a visitor?"

Both men ignored Jeremy's question. Dr. Becker shook the new arrival's hand.

Hebert said, "I'm truly sorry our regulations won't allow you to tour the laboratories with your son."

"We were hoping there'd be some way to get around that."

Jeremy said, "My chief was supposed to set it up this morning. Didn't he call your staff?"

"He did set it up, Jeremy." Hebert held out his hand. "May I call you Jeremy?"

"Sure." He shook Hebert's hand.

"But your chief didn't tell us your father is HIV-negative. Our legal staff is adamant about keeping anybody who's negative out of the working labs. The viruses we use are actually well contained, but you know how lawyers are—it's their job to protect us from liability."

"Out of curiosity," Dr. Becker said, "how did you learn I'm negative? I suspect you knew it before we got to that guard out front."

"You're right, we did. We have access to the national registry that stores information used by M-E-Ps all over the country. The PR people run a screen on all our visitors—it's a routine part of the clearance procedures."

Dr. Becker shrugged. "That's the second time in as many days I've been discriminated against because I don't have HIV."

Hebert smiled. "I'm sorry."

"Forget it. You didn't make the regulations. You fellows have a good tour. I'll see you back at the Infirmary, Jeremy—sometime in the late afternoon."

"You're sure you don't mind?" Jeremy asked. "I can do the tour some other time." He glanced at Hebert, looking for assurance that he could arrange a rain check. He was unnerved to find the man staring intently at him.

Dr. Becker shook his head. "No, no. You go ahead. I can use the time anyway—make some phone calls. Maybe even take a nap."

Hebert escorted both of them to the hallway at the rear of the briefing room where he said goodbye to Dr. Becker then led Jeremy down a corridor in the opposite direction.

"Tell me about yourself," Jeremy said. "You told us you work in Virology, what's your professional background?"

Hebert laughed, then grinned at Jeremy. "That's not part of the tour, but since it's you.... I am a virologist. I grew up south of here in Morgan City, then I started in pre-med at LSU. After a couple of years I realized medicine wasn't quite what I wanted, so I switched to basic sciences. My masters and PhD are both in microbiology—from Columbia."

Jeremy was surprised and his look must have shown it.

"What's the matter? Did I say something wrong?"

"No, not at all. I just didn't think a PhD virologist in a place like this would be a tour guide."

"We all do it in rotation. The boss says he likes to keep the professional staff in touch with the public."

"Something like hospital scut work," Jeremy mumbled. "Drawing blood, things like that."

"What did you say?" Hebert asked.

"Nothing important. I guess every job has its share of scut work." He looked at Hebert. "What happened after Columbia? How'd you end up in New Orleans?"

"I was a research associate at NIH for a while. I got interested in basic virus research and genetic engineering, and I was trying to work out a transfer into the Viral Disease Institute when the board recruited me to come down here as Chief of the Live Virus Section."

Jeremy raised his eyebrows. "Columbia, National Institutes of Health, now the Regional HIV Lab. Sounds like the fast track to me, Dr. Hebert."

A smile flitted across the man's face as he buttoned his lab coat. "Thanks, Jeremy. By the way, my name is Daniel—my friends call me Dan."

❖ ❖ ❖

26

The Keynote Address

Barbara had left Jeremy alone with his computer when he told her he was thinking about that man Guidry who'd become a thorn in their sides during their long ago years at Charity. He wasn't surprised when she left—she'd told him many times she thought of Guidry as her own personal demon and she didn't want to hear anything more about him.

Jeremy padded barefoot around his study as he tried to push those troublesome days at Charity out of his mind. He adjusted the belt of the tartan robe he wore over running clothes while working late at night on his keynote address for the World AIDS Conference. He'd already decided not to mention Guidry and the other bad actors from those years. The Conference didn't need to hear about those things anyway—better stick to the unfolding events that marked the tedious progress of researchers and physicians in the battle against the elusive HIV.

That's what they wanted to hear from him—how those years looked to an HIV-positive physician who'd lived through all the bright hopes and all the awful fears and disappointments. They wanted to hear about how the Health Protection Act had created a strangely artificial kind of segregation and how that law had influenced progress toward a cure—did it push research forward or hold it back? What had finally triggered the changes that came later? What was going on at the grass roots level during all those years? Those were the things he'd tell 'em about.

Jeremy sat down and pulled his yellow legal pad closer. He sharpened his #2 pencil, then began some preliminary notes about that futuristic HIV Research Facility he and his father had visited. He wanted his words to give the conference a visual picture of the place—not only what it looked like, but what it felt like to an ambitious young surgeon and to an older practitioner who'd experienced it first-hand. He wanted the folks at the conference to wonder, as he had wondered, why such generous appropriation of taxpayer monies had not been able to conquer the HIV—why it had not been able to end the spread of AIDS that still swept across the country like a barely controlled wildfire.

He decided to share the excitement of nomination for the Nobel Prize for Medicine, a great hope that came to the Research Facility and the leaders of its Virology Section who spearheaded development of the NOLA Strain. He'd summarize some of the ways their work influenced research in those years. Should he mention that virologist, Daniel Hebert, who'd toured him through the NOLA lab? Hebert was head man of the live virus labs. No, probably better to keep quiet about that part of it—Jeremy had later figured out Hebert's role at the Research Facility was a great deal more than head honcho of live viruses. He had influenced the progress of AIDS research in many ways more than just guiding the work of the Live Virus Section.

The early light of a cloudless October dawn brightened the windows of Jeremy's study by the time he finished the editing and re-editing of that part of his keynote speech. He pushed his chair back from the desk and walked to the kitchen to make a new pot of coffee before awakening Barbara to share it with him.

Early as it was, he'd decided to roust her out of bed anyway. He wanted more than a coffee companion. He was eager for Barbara to proofread his night's work on the speech. Like everything else in their marriage, she was a valued helpmate in developing the keynote address. She was very good at spotting what would click with the conference attendees and what would not, and she didn't mind telling him what she thought about what he'd written.

27

NOLA Strain

LEAVING HIS FATHER IN THE LOBBY OF THE HIV RESEARCH Facility, Jeremy followed Daniel Hebert in the opposite direction, down a long corridor then around the corner to a dead end. Hebert glanced up when he pressed the call button for an elevator. "If you don't mind, I'll give you some of our standard lecture as we go along."

"I don't mind at all," Jeremy said. "I'd like to hear it."

"Good. Stop me if I get too basic for you. Most of our visitors are medical laymen."

"I wondered about that."

"Right, most of the tours are set up by politicians trying to reassure their constituents that everything possible is being done to find a cure for AIDS—show them where some of their tax money is going."

"Yeah, that, too. I was gonna ask about the money. Don't you think that briefing room is a little plush for a public institution? Wouldn't the money do more good in research?"

"It's all political, Jeremy. Our funding is very generous."

"I agree with that. Two billion dollars every year for the research centers is a heavy load for the taxpayers on top of health care and everything else."

"Most people think of the money as an investment toward future reductions in health care costs, Jeremy."

"Maybe so, but I could do without some of that megabucks high tech stuff—all that's not helping anybody with AIDS."

Hebert smiled. "Every penny of that comes from construction funding—money we couldn't divert to research if we wanted to. It's locked up in accounts that can only be used for capital improvement."

Inside the elevator Jeremy noticed there were no buttons for selecting a floor. Instead, each floor number had two keyholes alongside it. Hebert took a pair of keys from his pocket and inserted them beside one of the numbers, a negative number. He turned both keys and the elevator moved down to a lower level where they walked into a small room with no other visible doors.

Hebert moved to the opposite wall and opened a small sliding panel to expose a security console. He inserted a bright yellow card that, except for its prominent color, resembled an M-E-P card. A lighted screen, much larger than the thumb-sized ones, blinked on the console, and Hebert placed his right hand against it. The terminal apparently read his entire hand print. A heavy steel door slid open without a sound.

Hebert led the way into a maze of corridors whose steel walls made the place look like some enormous bank vault. Jeremy saw no doors and wondered where they'd go from there. Then he noticed a series of narrow horizontal windows along each wall, and Hebert stopped at one of them. "This is our basic virology laboratory. It's like a factory—produces a steady supply of the HIV and other retroviruses for the entire facility."

Through the double plate glass window, Jeremy saw four workers inside the laboratory, each of them wearing long-sleeved white coveralls, white ankle boots, and white hoods. Protective goggles and breathing filters covered their faces and they all wore rubber gloves. With no part of their skin exposed, they looked more like robots than people.

"Do you worry about contamination?" Jeremy asked. "The workers look well protected, but what about the rest of us?"

"There's more than you can see. Each room has its own air control system."

"Temperature and humidity?"

Hebert nodded. "Right…air flow and pressure, too. Each lab is a self-contained environment with air locks for entering or leaving. The exhaust air is pumped through a series of filters that stop everything down to molecular size."

The tour continued down the steel corridor, stopping at several more laboratory windows where robot look-alikes were busy inside. "Impressive," Jeremy said. "Looks like some kind of orbital space ship."

He glanced at Hebert and caught him staring again. Hebert must have known he was spotted that time—he cut Jeremy a big smile.

They made several turns in the maze of corridors and peered into more labs, each one set up for a different specialized function. Finally they came to a break room and Hebert motioned Jeremy inside. Unlike the futuristic labs, the break room looked earth bound, like an ordinary coffee shop decorated in bright sunny colors with murals of out-of-doors open spaces on every wall—scenic mountains, wild rivers, grass filled prairies.

No robots in the break room either—half a dozen normal looking men and women sat at the tables, all of them wearing ordinary clothing. On the way to the coffee counter Hebert stopped beside one group and introduced Jeremy, but when they returned with steaming mugs Hebert made a point of choosing an empty table. "This'll give us a little more privacy," he said. "The others'll be going back to the labs in a couple of minutes anyway. They only get a short break."

Jeremy shrugged. "Fine with me." He sipped the hot coffee and looked around the room, impressed with its bright, sunlit feeling—then it hit him. The place smelled like newly mown grass and fragrant wildflowers. Damn, more construction funding for special effects.

Hebert put his mug down and asked, "How long have you been in the surgery program, Jeremy?"

"This is my fourth year."

"Fourth year...that's senior level, isn't it? With your own team?"

"That's right. We have two years as seniors, then a final year as chief resident."

"Pretty tough years, I hear."

Jeremy smiled. "It's steady—we're on duty every other night?"

"Where do you live? Outside the hospital, I mean?"

"I have an small apartment in the Quarter."

"In the Quarter? Where is it?"

"On Burgundy—three hundred block."

"You're married then?"

"No, I share the apartment with another surgery resident. We work on alternating nights, so we both use it as a getaway."

"Do you worry much about being HIV-positive before you even begin your practice?"

"You sound like my dad." He smiled, then hesitated.

What was Hebert up to, guiding their conversation to personal things like that? "No, I don't worry about it anymore—worrying doesn't change things, but I'm convinced it helps to stay busy. Besides, I'm counting on you guys in this lab making a discovery that'll give me a very long time to practice surgery."

"I believe that'll happen, Jeremy, but you have to keep it in perspective. Developing drugs to destroy the HIV without harming the patient is a tedious process. A few times we've thought we had a winner, but each drug that looked promising in the laboratory proved a lot less effective in living patients. Sometimes we run into unexpected toxicity, but more often the problem is drug resistance. Before the new drug has a chance to be effective, the virus undergoes natural mutation, making it resistant to a drug that looked great on the drawing board."

"Yeah. I've seen plenty of that in the clinical trials."

"Seems like every time we test a new drug the virus has already changed its fundamental biology. The traditional methods of developing effective drugs have turned into a bizarre kind of hide-and-seek with the genome of an evolving virus."

"Tell me about the NOLA strain. I read your press release—sounds like a pretty big discovery."

"It is big—may be the most important research tool to come along yet. You read about the Nobel nomination?"

Jeremy nodded and loosened his tie. The Nobel nomination was exciting all right, but it wasn't what he really wanted to know. "I hear the NOLA strain has led you to an experimental treatment plan that looks promising."

Hebert grinned. "We think it is. It looks damn good in the lab, and we're eager to get it into human trials. I have the privilege of being a principal investigator on this one."

"That's great. Tell me about it."

"It looks like we've found a way to slow down virus mutation—maybe stop it completely. The NOLA strain allowed us to complete the laboratory phase of that protocol in record time. Then, once our folks mapped the HIV genome, they were able to pinpoint the exact spot that regulates mutation."

"The specific gene, you mean?"

"That's right. Once the controlling gene was identified, we were able to produce it artificially by gene splicing in harmless bacteria. Then we changed the gene in ways the virus couldn't detect—reprogrammed its instructions to the virus. When the new gene is reimplanted the growing HIV accepts it, which means the virus can reproduce and it can infect, but it cannot change its genome. It can no longer mutate."

"But that wouldn't destroy the virus would it?"

"No, it's like we've put a governor on it. The more or less paralyzed virus then becomes a stationary target for some of the virus-killing drugs that have been around for a couple of years. The game of genetic hide-and-seek may soon be over."

"But you don't know if it'll actually work in the human body, do you?"

"No, we don't—that's where the clinical trials come in. Our plan is to introduce the synthetic gene into the blood stream of HIV-positive patients in hope that the natural viruses in their bodies will accept the modified gene. If that works, the modified viruses should reproduce themselves and very gradually replace the 'normal' ones." He signaled quotes for the word, normal, with his fingers. "Then mutation will stop, and the infection can be eliminated with a second drug. It's a kind of on-line genetic engineering in the body of an infected patient, like a one-two punch that causes the virus to stand still long enough to be hit by the drug that knocks it out."

"Sounds like exactly what I've been waiting for. What about protection for people who are still HIV-negative? Does it look like your protocol might lead to a vaccine—something to prevent new infections?"

"Not exactly a vaccine, Jeremy. Maybe something better. We believe the harmless bacteria that we've put to work producing the modified HIV gene can be colonized in the human intestinal tract. If we're right, the bacteria will live there forever, just waiting for an active HIV to come along. They'll produce an endless supply of the modified genetic protein, and any reproducing virus should accept it and become the less active strain. Then, if those patients become HIV-positive, they should respond quickly to treatment—new cases could be treated as soon as they're detected by a blood test. We could totally eliminate human AIDS in a few years."

"All right—I like the sound of that. How can we help you? What can we do at the hospital?"

Hebert glanced at his watch and stood up. "We need to get moving, Jeremy. I want to take you to the NOLA strain laboratory."

"Okay, but how can we help?"

"You can recruit patients," Hebert said. He bussed their coffee mugs then led Jeremy into the corridor. "You can recruit HIV-positive patients to volunteer as test subjects for the toxicity trials for our new protocol."

"Tell me what sort of patients you're looking for, I'll get the volunteers for you."

"That's a problem right now—I'm revising the criteria. We've tried to test the first part of the protocol, the part about implanting the modified virus genome, but it looks like we chose the wrong patients. Most of them died before we really got the testing started."

Jeremy looked at Hebert. "We've seen some unexpected deaths recently, maybe they're the same ones you're talking about. Can you get me the names of the patients you selected for the new protocol?"

Dan averted his glance. "The names are confidential, Jeremy—part of our agreement with the patients when they sign up for the volunteer pool. That's one thing I hope to change. I want to take the new protocol out of the volunteer pool. I've asked the Review Committee to approve selecting test subjects for this protocol according to more specific criteria, not from the pool."

"Just tell me about your selection criteria. We'll find the volunteers you need."

Still talking, Hebert urged Jeremy along the corridor at a brisk pace. "The full-fledged testing will involve a series of injections of bacteria containing the modified virus gene. We'll have to do frequent blood tests to determine the patients' responses and look for any side effects. Animal testing in the lab has not shown harmful side effects, so we're pretty optimistic about that. But we don't know whether we can actually modify the virus in a living patient."

"Don't worry, we can get the patients to volunteer. Most of 'em are as eager as we are to see a treatment breakthrough."

"Good, we'll count on that." Hebert did not slow down, and he did not respond to Jeremy's enthusiasm about the volunteers. They came to an apparent dead end where he opened another sliding panel and repeated the hand print ID routine, but this entry required a second level of confirmation. Hebert spoke into a recessed microphone and, after his voice pattern was verified, a steel door opened silently, operated by a mechanism so sophisticated it made the huge door appear weightless.

They passed through a small negative-pressure room which made Jeremy's ear's pop, then they scrubbed their hands and forearms and pulled on disposable coveralls and shoe covers and, finally, caps and masks. "This is the NOLA Lab," Hebert said, leading Jeremy inside.

The NOLA Laboratory contained equipment on the cutting edge of virology, some of it Jeremy had never even heard of. Hebert pointed out various robot-garbed technologists working at some of the benches, but Jeremy was stunned when he stopped at an ordinary looking wall safe. "That's where we store the living cultures of HIV, NOLA strain. Would you like to see them?"

"No, thanks," Jeremy replied, backing away from the safe. "I'll pass on that part of the tour."

Hebert smiled. "What's the matter?"

"That's not exactly the kind of storage place I expected for a potent virus like NOLA."

"It's actually very secure. But you're right about NOLA being potent. Conceivably it could be very dangerous."

"What would happen if the NOLA strain infected a human being?"

"We don't know, of course, because it's never happened. But remember, NOLA reproduces a thousand times faster than ordinary strains. It would probably cause a rapidly progressing illness that resembles AIDS. Moving that fast, I doubt if the disease could be controlled by any known treatment."

"That's what I mean about storing the virus in that safe. Is it really secure?"

"Don't worry about it. Like ordinary strains, NOLA can't survive very long outside the body. The safe has a heating system to maintain the interior at body temperature, but out here in the room the virus would die as soon as it cooled off—maybe half an hour."

"That makes sense, but what about sabotage? A terrorist could raise hell with that virus culture."

Hebert shrugged and made a palms-up gesture. "You've seen the security devices that separate this room from the rest of the lab. The entire underground section of the building is surrounded by sufficient shielding to resist any known explosive device. We believe it's impossible to enter these labs without prior authorization."

Jeremy pretended to be more reassured than he actually was, but he kept his distance from the wall safe. He fought to contain his enthusiasm as they left the NOLA area. He'd been to the mountain. He knew a cure for AIDS could come out of these laboratories—and, with it, the end of the segregated lifestyle he and many others had been squeezed into by the Health Protection Act. "I'm eager to tell the other residents about your protocol," he said. "They'll want to sign up all their patients as soon as you give me the new criteria for test subjects."

Daniel stopped and drew Jeremy aside. "Listen, we're not prepared to test a large number of patients at one time, at least not at first. We need to keep the numbers fairly small because of all the testing we have to do on each patient. I'd rather start out with all of the patients from one service. You might even be able to get enough volunteers from your team alone."

Jeremy frowned. "I don't understand. I thought...."

"You'll be out of town for a week, right?"

How in the hell did Hebert know about that? "Well, yes, I'm going home with my dad."

"I'll try to have the new criteria ready by the time you get back." He pulled out his wallet. "Here's my card, Jeremy. Call me when you're back at work and we can set up a plan for your team to be the clearing house for our volunteers."

Had he mentioned leaving town? If he had, he sure couldn't remember it. He took the card from Hebert and looked at it. "Assistant Chairman, Virology Department? You didn't tell me that. I thought you were a section head."

Hebert grinned. "I fill both slots, actually, but the Live Virus Section is what I like. That's where the action is."

After saying goodbye, Jeremy negotiated the security checkpoints to leave the building and walked into the noise and exhaust fumes of late afternoon traffic. It was the longest time he'd been out of bed since his head injury, and he was not surprised when the clamor and the stink triggered a pounding headache.

The pain distracted him, but he couldn't get rid of a nagging worry about Daniel Hebert. The guy had seemed eager to move quickly into full-fledged testing of his new protocol, then he did a three-sixty and wanted to limit it to a smaller group. Why? Why would he want all of the volunteers to be from one hospital team? Why not enroll 'em throughout the hospital? Seemed like that'd be a lot quicker, even if they couldn't test 'em all at once.

28

Beaumont

By mid-morning on Friday Jeremy and his father were driving west out of New Orleans on Interstate 10. Skirting the western edge of Lake Ponchatrain, the highway crossed marshy wetlands with cypress trees and cattails, then followed the Mississippi River upstream through higher plains of sandy loam. Loblolly pines lined the road, almost as thick as the sugar cane growing in fields nearby. By the time they reached Baton Rouge Jeremy had gone over every detail of his lab tour with Daniel Hebert.

"Sounds like he impressed you," Dr. Becker said. "Do you really think that double barreled treatment plan's as good as he says?"

"I'm convinced it is." Jeremy glanced up, hoping for some echo of his own confidence. Why had he never gotten a single positive comment about AIDS treatments from his father? Not one encouraging word. He usually said nothing, or changed the subject—acted like he thought HIV disease was invariably fatal and nothing would ever change that. Intellectually he had to know better, but emotionally.... He acted like he'd never stopped grieving after Jeremy became HIV-positive, grieving for an impending death that Jeremy was determined would not happen.

"What's Hebert's position at the lab, anyway? Did he say?"

"I asked him—he heads one of the virus labs. He's also assistant chief of the Virology Department."

"Not bad. He's a young man, too. What, thirty-five maybe?"

Jeremy nodded. "About that."

"Is he from this part of the country?"

"He said he grew up in Morgan City. He was an undergrad at LSU."

"Good. Wonder how he got such a high-powered job?"

"Probably good at what he does. He was at NIH before." Jeremy rearranged the rolled sweater he was using for a pillow. He couldn't get Hebert out of his mind—couldn't forget the way the guy kept staring at him. He'd seen that look a few times before, from gay men coming on to him. Could that be it? No matter—he didn't expect to see Hebert again.

Later they stopped for lunch in Lake Charles, then crossed the Sabine River and entered eastern Texas. Driving into Beaumont by mid-afternoon, they left the highway at Eleventh Street. Then, just north of the restored Old Town, they turned on Long Avenue and drove into a high-end district of large older homes. In its early years the neighborhood had been deliberately sited far away from the hustle and bustle of Gladys City's oil well, a long way from the noise of the sawmills and the dangers respectable citizens imagined around the Port of Beaumont on the Neches River.

The Becker home was a two-story red brick Tudor with exposed half-timbers. The parking court and both garages at the rear of the house were empty when they arrived. Retrieving the luggage, Dr. Becker held the back door open for Jeremy. "I don't like that headache you had last night. Why don't you lie down for a while."

"Okay, I do feel a little tired. You probably want to call the office anyway, don't you?" He turned back at the foot of the stairs. "Let me know when Mom gets here."

Entering his old room was a trip backward in time, a trip to the warm memories of high school and earlier days when he and his sister, Elaine, had grown up in the embrace of a loving family in this grand old home. Swimming trophies from high school were still displayed on the bookcase, mixed among his favorite books and collections of things. Several yearbooks were stacked beneath a large scrapbook Jeremy had never completed. Framed pictures of each year's swimming team and certificates for outstanding performances hung on the walls.

He took his senior yearbook from the shelf before stretching out on the bed and flipped to a double-page spread of snapshots. God, did he ever really look like that? There's ol' Matt…and who's that guy on the.... He fell asleep before turning the page.

The familiar smell of searing roast beef triggered a brief dream in which Jeremy awakened from exhausted sleep after a four-hour swimming practice. That aroma could only mean one thing—his mom was home. He rushed down the stairs, then stood without speaking at the kitchen door. Just stood there admiring his mother.

Born Catherine Morrison, she had grown up in a close-knit, working class family in New Orleans. After earning her master's degree in public relations she had taken a position at Tulane, where she met the handsome, red-haired medical student from Minnesota who later became her husband.

When the couple came to Beaumont, Catherine Becker had kept in touch with her public relations background by part-time consulting at a local radio station and for the county medical society. Now, in her fifties, she remained an attractive woman who appeared ten years younger. She turned from the stove, saw her son and threw her arms open. "Jeremy! How are you, baby? I've really been worried about you. What a horrible thing to happen—those people beating you."

He walked into her embrace, still unaccustomed to being taller. "I'm okay, Mom. At least it gave me a good reason to spend a few days with you and Dad."

Hugging him close, she continued, "I'm so glad to see you. Your father told me you were all right, but you know me. I have to see for myself." She fingered through his thick blond hair like a grooming primate. "How's that cut? Oh, my God, it's so big! What did they hit you with?"

Jeremy moved away from her searching fingers. "It was only their fists, Mom. Could have been a ring, I guess. Anyway it's about healed now, so it doesn't matter."

"You doctors. I think it's awful." She kept her arm linked through his and guided him to a stool at the breakfast bar. "Sit down. Talk to me while I fix supper." A smile teased the corners of her eyes. "I thought you might like a pot roast."

"You know it's my favorite. It smells wonderful."

They spent the next half hour catching up on family news and Jeremy's progress in his residency. Finally, Jeremy reached for his mother's hands and toyed with her wedding ring. "Mom, I invited a friend to come from New Orleans for a few days next week." He looked up and watched Catherine's face. "Her name's Barbara Allison. She's a nurse on the cardiology ward, a good friend who's been especially nice to me while I was in the hospital. We've been going out for a while."

She nodded and gave his hand a reassuring pat. "That's fine, Jeremy. Your father told me about Barbara. I look forward to meeting her." She kissed her son on the forehead. "Barbara can stay in Elaine's room."

"Elaine's room?" He smiled and slipped his arm around her waist. "I'd hoped Elaine might come home for the weekend. Anyway, Barbara's my guest, Mom. We don't need to use Elaine's room."

"Elaine's busy at school this weekend." Catherine said nothing more…she just turned away and busied herself with adding vegetables to the pot roast. Jeremy knew that was all he'd get. He knew she'd just agreed to Barbara's sharing his room, and he knew she would not bring it up again.

The following Tuesday Jeremy drove to the airport to meet Barbara's arriving flight. When she walked from the passenger gate he felt a rush of pure joy, and the two of them came together in an unplanned embrace. "How're you doing?" she asked. "Any more headaches?"

"No. I'm fine. Really fine now that you're here." Beaming, he took her hand and headed for the luggage pickup.

As they loaded her things into the car, conversation turned to the hospital. "I brought some notes from Joe," Barbara said. We put together a list of the patients who've died, and Joe reviewed their hospital records. Six of 'em altogether."

Jeremy shook his head and slipped behind the steering wheel. "Anything new in the medical records?"

"I don't know—Joe didn't have time to talk about it. He gave me his notes just before I left for the airport."

"When did he decide to review the records? Must have been a last-minute thing."

"No. He was supposed to finish it earlier, but he had trouble getting the records. They were all in an administrative secure file, risk management or something. Joe had to get...what's his name? In Education...Hollander. He had to ask Dr. Hollander to get him an authorization from Mr. Lockhart to review the charts."

"Secure file? That's odd—I've never run into that."

Jeremy pulled his mother's car out of the airport and headed to Cardinal Drive, then past Lamar University and the Spindletop Museum. "What's that campus?" Barbara asked. "I didn't know there was a college in Beaumont."

"Lamar University. Something like sixteen thousand students." He pointed to a tall gray obelisk. "See that granite monument over there, on the edge of the campus?"

"Yes. It's huge. What on earth is it?"

"That's the Lucas Gusher Monument."

"Is this a joke, Jeremy? What's a Lucas Gusher?"

"No joke. It's a national landmark—the exact spot that made Beaumont a boomtown."

"Oh, really? Tell me about it."

"This whole area was an oil field called Spindletop. A huge gusher blew in right there in 1901. January tenth. It sprayed oil a couple of hundred feet into the air for about ten days before anybody could cap it. Three quarters of a million barrels of crude oil flooded this whole area."

"I think I heard about that in school. How'd they clean it up?"

"The oil burned a couple of months later—sparks from some locomotive set it off. Poor old Lucas didn't make much money from his gusher. The well never produced much after he capped it, but it was the beginning of the oil industry in Texas."

Barbara gave his leg a squeeze. "Sounds like a Texas tall tale to me."

"God's truth," he said, grinning.

Catherine was waiting when they reached the house, and Jeremy relaxed while she and Barbara got to know each other. Alike in many ways, they were both self-confident career women who had succeeded at working alongside men as intellectual equals.

Later, after dinner, they all decided to go over Joe's notes from the chart reviews, and Barbara brought the thick folder to Dr. Becker's study. "Joe told me all of the patients were recovering from whatever illness brought 'em to the hospital in the first place," she said. "All of 'em were HIV-positive, of course, but Joe said none of them had any sign of AIDS. Each patient had volunteered for one of the treatment protocols from the research lab."

They went over Joe's notes line by line and discovered a few more similarities. Each of the unfortunate patients had a blood count of helper T-cells in excess of five hundred one or two days prior to death, and that was normal. But four of them had repeat counts of less than a hundred during the final hours of their lives. Most of them, for one reason or another, had blood cultures collected a short time before they died, but none of the cultures grew any bacteria.

Every one of the patients seemed to be doing well before they suddenly developed high fever, then delirium, finally deep coma. All of them had rapid heart rates and falling blood pressure. In each case, the residents treated the shock aggressively, but none of the patients showed any response. Each one died within a few hours after the onset of that sudden turn for the worse.

Quiet during the review, Dr. Becker finally spoke, to no one in particular. "So similar—all six deaths." He shook his head. "Doesn't sound like natural causes to me. Something's not right about all this, but what is it? Clinically it doesn't make sense. Is it some kind of foul play?"

Jeremy avoided telling his father about Joe's problem getting the dead patients' charts. No use getting him excited about the front office again. "I agree," he said. "It's way too much to be coincidence. Let's telephone Joe. He could take his reviews to Lockhart in the morning. Tell him what we're worried about."

"No," Dr. Becker said. "Not Lockhart. My feelings about that administrator have not changed. I'm convinced we can't trust the man."

Jeremy put his hand on his father's arm. "I know you don't like Lockhart, but we've got to get somebody in authority involved. We're getting in over our heads here."

Barbara and Catherine agreed. Experienced at relieving the tense moods her husband's vociferous opinions could create, Catherine said, "I feel left out here. No medical background, remember? What do those blood counts mean?"

"They were normal at first," Barbara said, "then they fell to dangerously low levels."

"The helper T-cells are critical in the body's immune responses," Jeremy added.

Catherine's public relations training came through. "We'd better be careful with this." She moved behind her husband's chair and massaged his shoulders. "You said we only have suspicions at this point—you know how quickly innocent people can become headline fodder. A suggestion, a question to the wrong person could result in unintended damage."

"Okay, we'll be careful," Dr. Becker said. He patted one of her massaging hands. "But we can't just let it drop. I agree with Jeremy—we need to involve somebody who can do something. Suppose I telephone Warren Randall in the morning?"

"Who's Randall," Barbara asked.

"Warren Randall is one of our U.S. Senators, Barbara. He's from Beaumont, and he's been in the Senate long enough to get some fairly senior appointments. He was just beginning his political career when I opened my practice, and he became both my patient and a good friend. Our families used to vacation together. We've stayed in touch over the years, so I feel comfortable discussing this with him."

Jeremy objected. "Dad, how can Senator Randall help us? None of this is happening in Texas."

"Warren's Chairman of the Senate Judiciary Committee, Jere. He's bound to have a working relationship with the Justice Department, with the FBI. His staff helped pass the Health Protection Act. They got the Senate to support funding for the regional HIV labs. You know how close your hospital is to the whole business of HIV legislation—Warren would want to know about the deaths."

They all agreed with that logic, and Dr. Becker took his wife's hand. "Maybe he'll believe the whole thing is some silly fantasy, but I don't think so." He turned to Jeremy. "I'll try to reach him at home in the morning—before he goes to work."

Catherine gave his hand a squeeze and kissed him on the cheek. "Great idea, sweetheart. Warren'll help us if he thinks we have a problem." She glanced at Jeremy with a familiar look and a wink that said the senator would keep the whole thing under control. He wouldn't let their concerns blow it out of proportion.

The conversation drifted to Beaumont politics, and Jeremy grew restless. With a furtive glance at Barbara, he got up to leave the room, saying he wanted to take a shower. He finished the shower in record time, then slipped on a soft terry robe. Sitting in his room, feet propped on one of the twin beds, he opened a well-worn edition of Benét's *John Brown's Body* to read a few of his favorite passages.

Something touched his forehead, something soft. He opened his eyes—the room was dark, lighted only from the bathroom. He smiled when he saw it was Barbara, smelling clean and damp from her own shower, wearing a short, pale yellow nightgown.

"I hate to wake you up," she said, "but you look mighty uncomfortable." She combed the hair back from his forehead with her fingers. "Which bed is mine?"

He found her hand and pulled her down on his lap. "Which bed do you want?"

"Doesn't matter."

"Take your pick. Either one, you have to share it with me."

"Oh, do I now?" She slipped her hand inside his robe and teased his bare chest.

Later, Barbara nudged away from him in their shared bed. They hovered together in that magic space between sleeping and waking, savoring the close bond that had grown between them. He kissed her softly, and she turned her body to nest in his warm curve. He kissed her on the back of the neck, and whispered, "I love you, Barbara."

❖❖❖

29

THE SENATOR

AT SIX-FIFTEEN THE FOLLOWING MORNING JEREMY'S FATHER returned to his study and dialed Senator Randall's home number in Washington. He knew enough about Randall's schedule to be certain of the best time to catch him. The senator's wife answered the telephone.

"Good morning, Beth. This is David Becker. Hope I didn't wake you."

"No, no, we've been up for a while. How are you, David? How's the family?"

"We're all fine. Jeremy's recovering fast. I guess you heard what happened to him?"

"Yes, we read about it. Warren takes *The Times-Picayune.* I couldn't believe it when he showed me the article. Outrageous—those people beating him up like that."

"I think he'll be okay. He's with us in Beaumont for a few days." He glanced at the grandfather clock standing near the door. "Listen, I need to speak to Warren if he's still there."

"He's right here—I'll put him on. Give my love to Catherine and the children."

Senator Randall's voice came on the line. "Good morning, David. Good timing. Another ten minutes and I'd have been on the beltway. What can I do for you?"

Dr. Becker told him of the unexpected deaths at Charity and Jeremy's assault by the family of one of the dead patients.

"What does the hospital administration think about it?"

"That's the problem. The administrator at Charity is the most unreasonable man I've ever tried to deal with. Downright obstructive, if you ask me. Like he's trying to cover up something. The whole thing doesn't sit right with me, Warren. I'm worried about some kind of foul play."

The senator laughed. "You always have liked a good mystery, haven't you? Remember that summer at Lake Texoma when you insisted I read three of your Agatha Christies?"

"Warren, this is not fiction. I'm worried about Jeremy and the rest of the hospital staff, and I'm worried about the reputation of the hospital itself. Surely you can appreciate the potential damage to public support for the Regional HIV Lab. Don't forget, that's your pet project."

"Hey, calm down, old friend. Just giving you a hard time. All the patients must be HIV-positive. How do you know they didn't die of AIDS?"

"Come on, Warren. None of them had the least indication of AIDS. They were all hospitalized for different reasons. Anyway, AIDS couldn't possibly cause them to die that quickly."

"Okay, okay. I believe you. I admit it sounds like too many similar events to be coincidence."

A long silence on the line convinced Dr. Becker the senator needed time to develop a plan. Probably cooking up some way to satisfy a fairly influential constituent without getting too deeply involved.

"Tell you what I'll do," the senator said finally. "I plan to be in Beaumont for several days at the end of next week. I'll ask around before I come home—see what I can find out. Let's get together in Beaumont and go over the whole thing in detail."

Dr. Becker thought he was getting a congressional run-around.

"It'll be better if my visible involvement comes from Beaumont," Senator Randall said. "Louisiana is not my constituency, you know, so I need to be fairly discrete."

Dr. Becker knew his friend was intrigued, but he was disappointed by what he felt to be a low level of interest. "Good, Warren," he said. "Thanks. Call me if there's anything we can do from this end. I look forward to seeing you when you get to Beaumont."

Mulling over the senator's words, he went to the kitchen to make a cup of coffee. To his surprise, the others were waiting for him, and they all spoke at once.

"What did Warren say?" Catherine asked.

"What did the senator think?"

"What'd he tell you, Dad?"

"Wait a minute—I can only answer one question at a time."

Catherine handed him a cup of coffee. "Don't tantalize us. We're all eager to know what Warren thought."

With a little smile, he took a long sip of his coffee. Jeremy rolled his eyes toward the ceiling, and Barbara laughed at the two of them.

"Actually, I'm a little disappointed," he said. "Warren didn't sound very concerned. He laughed at first, embarrassed me really, but he did agree to ask a few questions—and to talk about it when he's here next week."

"Don't be disappointed," Jeremy said. "He agreed to check it out. That can mean a pretty thorough investigation."

"I know, but—"

"That's enough for me," Catherine said, hugging her husband. "Warren'll find out whether we need to be worried about all this. There's not another thing we can do until we hear from him, so let's all just stop fretting about it." She looked at the others. "I want us to enjoy Barbara and Jeremy's visit, so promise me you'll all stop playing detective."

❖

A few hours later, Jeremy and Barbara were laughing at old yearbooks in his bedroom when Catherine walked through the open door. "How nice to hear laughter from this room again. It's been a long time...so much has happened."

Jeremy hugged his mother. He knew she meant more than a few years passing. His HIV conversion had changed her life, too. Now she always seemed to tiptoe around him, like she was unwilling to disturb whatever remained of his life. Dammit...why? Why did it have to be like that? Shifting his mood, he grinned and gave her another squeeze. "Nothing's really changed, Mom. You look exactly the same as you did when I laughed in this room every single day."

"Thank you, Jeremy." She smiled and turned to Barbara. "Isn't he sweet?"

"I think he is." Barbara pointed to the yearbooks and grinned at Jeremy. "From the looks of those pictures, I'd say he's always been a sweet boy."

"Wait just a minute," Jeremy protested. "There's no way you could—"

"You wait a minute," Catherine said. "I came up here to invite you both to lunch at the Beaumont Club. Feel up to it?"

"Can we go to the Beaumont Club?" Jeremy asked. "Isn't the club segregated?"

"Not the restaurant. The pool and the fitness center are segregated, but not the restaurant."

Jeremy knew what she was doing—she wanted to introduce Barbara to some of her own friends who would just happen to be at the club for lunch on the same day.

He was right. Catherine's friends were waiting when they arrived at the downtown Beaumont Club. The three women sat near a large window, watching every new arrival with great curiosity while pretending not to notice. Each of them was dressed with casual elegance, make-up and hair whispering understatement, their presence plainly not an accident.

The Beaumont Club had a seventy-five year tradition of serving distinctive meals for Beaumont's elite. Its large rooms were warm and quiet, reeking of old elegance. Dark wood paneling and a rich mixture of long-polished brass and sparkling crystal surrounded sedate furnishings and an impressive collection of European landscape paintings. The faint aroma of a buttery sauté hung in the air.

Catherine spotted the other women immediately. "Jeremy, look who's here," she said. "Go over there and introduce Barbara to our friends. I'll ask Tony to give us a larger table so they can join us."

He smiled and went along with his mother's ruse, but as he led Barbara toward the group at the window he said, "I haven't seen these women in years, but they're my mother's closest friends. I'm pretty sure she set this up so they could meet you."

"That's sweet of her," Barbara said, then glanced at Jeremy. "Don't worry about it—mothers like to do that sort of thing."

The three women remained seated as they approached. One of them said, "Why, Jeremy Becker. What a nice surprise. I'm so glad to see you're recovering from that...that mean attack."

"Thank you, Mrs. Heath. You're looking well yourself." Jeremy bent down to kiss her on the cheek like he had always done, but she drew back and took him by the hand instead. Her rebuff caught him off guard. AIDS. He'd forgotten how rigid small town attitudes could be.

Finally Mrs. Heath asked, "And who's this with you?"

He brought Barbara into the group. "This is Barbara Allison. Barbara I'd like you to meet some family friends. This is Margaret Heath." He gestured to each of the women as he spoke. "Mary Alice Lattimer, Olivia McElhaney. Barbara Allison."

This time Jeremy was smart enough not to get too close. No more kisses. After a round of discrete hand shaking he and Barbara sat on a small sofa opposite the three women. "Barbara's a friend from New

Orleans," Jeremy said. "She was nice enough to come to Beaumont for a few days while I'm here." He winked broadly at Barbara for the benefit of the others. "These ladies have a lot to say about things that happen in Beaumont."

Olivia McElhaney protested. "Jeremy, stop teasing. You know that's not true. We're just interested in what's best for our town."

The others nodded their agreement. Olivia continued, "Barbara, we are so glad to have you here. Catherine told me you're a nurse. You must find that rewarding—where do you work?

"I'm at Charity, in the cardiology unit."

The three women glanced at each other.

"Charity?" Olivia said. "I thought Charity was the, uh, the infected hospital."

"It is," Jeremy said. "They call it the Medical Center of Louisiana now, and it is an HIV-positive hospital."

"I see.... Well, Barbara, does your family live in New Orleans?"

Before she could answer, Catherine arrived. "I see you've all met our house guest. Isn't she pretty?" She sat next to Barbara and gave her a hug. Smiling at her three friends, she said, "I've arranged a larger table so we can all have lunch together."

"Wonderful! Good idea, Catherine."

The women's duplicity gnawed at Jeremy. He took Barbara's hand, eager to get her out of there, but he knew they'd stay for his mother's sake.

"What a treat," Mary Alice Lattimer said, "to have lunch with Beaumont's dashing young doctor and his pretty nurse." Barbara laughed and Catherine beamed with pride.

Seething, Jeremy hoped Barbara missed the nuances of what the women were doing. At the table he was sure the three orchestrated the seating so that none of them sat beside him or Barbara.

During lunch Barbara was clearly the guest of honor, but the women continued their deft probing into her background. Polite but persistent, they learned everything she would tell them about her childhood and her family, about her education and her career.

When they left the Beaumont Club, Jeremy and Barbara drove Catherine to Radio Station KZZB for her afternoon's work as the station's public relations consultant, then continued past some of the town's sights. As they passed the Neches River waterfront Barbara said, "I had no idea there was a port for seagoing vessels in the middle of Texas."

Jeremy put his arm around her shoulders. "Not exactly the middle, but we do like to do things big. And we're full of surprises."

"I learned about that at lunch."

He turned to face her. "I'm sorry about that, Barbara. My mother can be pretty sneaky when it comes to getting her way."

"Don't worry about it, Jeremy. It's not a problem. Southern women are famous for that sort of thing." After a moment's thought she continued, "Actually, the same thing happens in Pennsylvania. You'd be the one in the hot seat if we visited my family."

He smiled and kissed her hand. "Okay, I'll remember that. But, something else is bothering me, Barbara. Something I can't get out of my mind."

"What are you talking about? Something to do with the deaths at the hospital?"

"Yes....I don't know. Maybe, but I really don't know. I just can't get it out of my mind." He raised his eyebrows and looked at her. "I'm worried about the lab techs drawing blood on those patients. We talked about it in the hospital, remember? But I don't think it stuck with my dad. I don't think he even mentioned it to Senator Randall."

She put her hands on his arm. "Why do you think that's so important, Jeremy?"

"You must know something's wrong about it. You know how hard it is to get anybody from the lab to come to the wards and draw blood."

She nodded. "You're right about that. What do you think it means?"

"I'm not sure yet. I think I'll ask Joe to help me snoop around the lab. Maybe we'll discover something."

"Why don't you just tell your father about it again. Let the senator's investigation check it out."

No, it may not mean anything. I want to be a more certain before I involve the senator. No use to make him look foolish if it turns out to be a wild goose chase."

"Why, Jeremy? Why does it have to be you checking it out?" Her face flushed. "You're just being stubborn. Why can't you tell the others about it?"

He looked at his watch, then squeezed her hand and turned a corner. "Barbara, a senate inquiry creates a mountain of paper work. It could tip off the wrong people that somebody's suspicious. Trust me on this one—I need your help."

"Well...okay. But just because it's you." She smiled and kissed his cheek. They drove home in silence, not angry silence, just nagging worry.

A steadily increasing sense of intimacy grew between them during the drive. Their hands found each other again, and no conversation was necessary. By the time they reached the house Jeremy sensed Barbara's arousal was as strong as his own. He led her up the stairs into his room and turned on a bedside radio. A rich Borodin melody filled the room as Jeremy drew her into his embrace and whispered, "I need you in my life, Barbara. I need you all the time. I love you, I truly love you. But dammit, I hate it that the HIV has to be a part of our future."

She kissed him gently. "I know. I used to get mad about that, too, but there's nothing we can do about it."

"You're right. We're both screwed up by things we couldn't do anything about. Me by a needle stick, you by that crazy kid you married." Jeremy kissed her eyelids. "You know we can't think about children. This damn virus is a heavy sentence to pass on to somebody you love."

"So?"

"I don't feel like I can ask you to marry me with that hanging over our heads."

"Don't worry about it." She stroked his beard. "There's plenty of time to get married. There'll be a cure before long—you told me how promising some of the new protocols are. We can talk about children after we get rid of the virus."

"You're incredible." He looked deeply into her brown eyes and shook his head. "God, I hope you're right about the cure."

During the days that followed it was apparent throughout the Becker household that Jeremy and Barbara were more than just casual friends. The elder Beckers silently approved. On Monday morning Jeremy walked into the kitchen as his mother was saying to Barbara, "...so happy. We like you very much, Barbara, and we hope he'll make you happy, too."

"Hi, Mom." He smiled at Barbara and took her hand. "I'm glad you approve."

"Good morning, Jeremy," Catherine said. "Don't worry about our woman talk. It's not for men's ears." She squeezed Barbara's other hand and kissed Jeremy on the cheek. "Your father called from the office. He'll be here at eleven to take you the airport."

Jeremy and Barbara said goodbye to Catherine at home—she was not going to the airport. Barbara said, "Be sure to tell Elaine I'm sorry I didn't get to meet her this time."

During the drive Dr. Becker told them Senator Randall had called him at the office.

"That's great, Dad" Jeremy said. "Why didn't you say something earlier?"

"I didn't want to worry your mother with it. She's not happy about you two being involved in all of this."

"What did the senator say, anyway? Has he learned anything new?"

"He wouldn't say much on the telephone, but he told me he'd uncovered something unusual. He wants to get together as soon as he gets to Beaumont. I'm going out to their house Friday night."

"He didn't say anything more?" Barbara asked. "Not even a hint about what he's discovered?"

"No, nothing. Said it's too soon. The main reason he called today was to tell me you two should not discuss our suspicions with anybody in New Orleans."

"What about Joe? He's already involved."

"Okay. Joe. But nobody else—especially nobody else at the hospital."

❖❖❖

30

BARBARA'S TALE

THE FLIGHT FROM BEAUMONT TO NEW ORLEANS WAS A SHORT one. Barbara gazed from the airplane's window as Jeremy's home town faded over the horizon. She liked his family and their friends, but they weren't the same as her own people.

They were all different people in a very different place from her own home town of Butler in western Pennsylvania. But the Beaumont women really wanted the same kind of reassurances her own mother had wanted. Barbara knew those women never realized she'd told them what she wanted them to know and not one thing more. She'd told the truth, but she didn't tell them one word more than they needed to know.

She slipped her arm through Jeremy's. "I want to tell you a story, Jere."

Jeremy opened his eyes and smiled. "What kind of story, love?"

"A story about your mother's friends and me—about me and my family in Butler." She shifted in her seat and turned toward Jeremy. "The women I met in Beaumont are so different from my own family and the friends I grew up with…." She smiled. "I can't tell you how many times I sat with a noisy group of women in my mother's kitchen in Pennsylvania. The women always gathered in our kitchen to gossip about others who weren't there or, sometimes, to complain about their husbands. They weren't elegant women like the ones in Beaumont. They were hard-working housewives with fat, blue-collar husbands and way too many children. One snowy Saturday morning during my senior year in high school I waited in that warm kitchen for the women to leave, waited for a chance to be alone with my mother."

"Why?" Jeremy asked. "Why did you wait for the others to leave?

Sounds like they were all your close friends."

"They were, but I wanted to have a serious talk with my mother. Finally, the women left in a flurry of snow boots, hand-knit mufflers, and matching hats. I screwed up all my courage, then hugged my mother's big waist and said, 'Mom, Scotty wants to get married.'"

"Mama pushed me away to arm's length and looked right into my face. 'Barbara,' she said, 'Scott's a nice boy. I know he loves you, but both of you are so young. Is that really what you want, darling?'"

"It is, Mama." I remember laying my head on her chest, and saying, "I really do love Scott."

"After that Mama sat me down at the kitchen table. She took a sip of her coffee and put the cup down. She wiped her hands on a dish towel then leaned over and took me by the shoulders. 'Barbara,' she said, 'I want you to be honest with me now. Are you pregnant?'"

"No, Mama! I'm not pregnant! We don't even plan to have a baby for a long time after we get married."

"That's a good idea, but what about the rest of it? You have to live, you know. It's true you'll both graduate in a few months, but what about your scholarship to nursing school?"

"I can still go to nursing school. Scotty knows a man who'll help him find a job in Philadelphia. We won't need much money—just the two of us."

"Barbara, Scott should be going to college himself."

"We talked about that. He'd rather work at first. I'll have a good job when I'm a nurse. He can go to college then if he wants to."

Barbara and Scott Allison got married two weeks after their high school graduation. They did go to Philadelphia, and Barbara entered nursing school, but the marriage had no chance of succeeding. They did all right for a year, then Scott decided he didn't really want a wife, and Barbara did want a career in nursing. They tried for nearly another year to work things out, but Scott drifted away into the convoluted world of closeted bisexuality and drug abuse, and they finally agreed divorce was the only way out. After the divorce Barbara never saw Scott again.

"You never told me all that," Jeremy said.

"Do you hate me for it?"

"Course not, I love you all the more for being a human being." He kissed her hand. "What became of Scott? Have you heard anything more from him?"

"No, not directly. I think he stayed in Philadelphia. Mama told me one of her friends heard he died of AIDS sometime in the early 80s."

"How do you feel about it now?" Jeremy asked. "Any regrets?"

"Regrets? Not really…." she grinned. "Nothing to regret except his unwanted gift of the HIV. I was too young to know what I was doing, that's all. Anyway, that's water under the bridge now. It's a different world, Jeremy, and we both have different lives to get on with, don't we?"

31

Back to Business

Jeremy's first day back at the hospital was a busy one. After early ward rounds with his team, he helped the junior residents with two hernia repairs, then assisted the attending staff with removal of a patient's cancerous stomach.

He would not again perform surgery himself, as primary surgeon, until he'd spent two or three days getting back into the rhythms of the team. That suited Jeremy. He knew the whole team's interactions were critical in the operating room, like those of a finely tuned orchestra. Even so, he was shocked to discover just how clumsy he felt after being away for only two weeks. But, much like riding a bicycle, the trained neural pathways that allowed his brain and muscles to work smoothly together were quickly reopened. By the end of the day's procedures he began to feel like himself again.

Richard Macleod, the chief resident, joined the team for evening rounds, catching up with them at a patient's bedside. "Hey, Jeremy. Good to see you back with the team. How're you doing?"

"Fine, Rich. I feel okay." He glanced at the others. "But I'm really out of shape. These guys are wearing me out."

"I know what you mean," Macleod said. "I noticed the same thing after I had my appendix out."

Later, he drew Jeremy aside. "Listen, I know your team's on call tonight. Would you rather take the night off? I could cover for you."

"No, no, I'm all right." He grinned and shoved his hands into the pockets of his hospital coat. "Thanks, anyway. In this rat race, it's nice to know somebody cares."

"No problem. We have to look after each other around here—you know that. Have to stay busy to keep ahead of the damn HIV." Macleod shook his head, then paused and looked at Jeremy. "Two interns on medicine had to drop out last month. Both of 'em had full-blown AIDS. Be sure to let me know if I can help you get up to speed. Take it easy for a while—don't push yourself too hard."

"Thank you, Rich. I'll let you know. Tonight's okay, though. Joe told me he'll be in the hospital tonight. If things get too hectic he'll bail me out."

After rounds Jeremy had supper with his team in the staff dining room, then went to the fourteenth floor for a nap. The night ahead could easily become a long one, and he wanted to pace himself.

Joe was in the room, reading at his desk. He looked tired, almost haggard. "How're you feeling, Joe? I bet you've been running yourself ragged, covering two teams while I was gone."

Joe shrugged. "Yeah, I was pretty busy. Not too bad though—the chief residents helped a lot."

"Macleod?"

"Yeah, he was the best, but both of 'em helped me a lot."

"Hey, I'm really sorry I did that to you."

"Sorry? What could you do about it? I'm just glad you're okay. A head injury's not the best way to start a career in surgery." Joe picked up the residents' call schedule from the desk. "I see we're both off tomorrow night. Let's have dinner somewhere. I'd like to hear what your father thought about the chart reviews I sent to Beaumont."

"Oh my god, Joe, I'm really sorry about that. I meant to fill you in as soon as I got back. We haven't been in the same place long enough to talk about much of anything."

"No, we haven't. I guess you've been pretty busy with Barbara and all. Did she make a hit with your family?"

Jeremy broke into a broad grin. "You know she did. She's great." He hesitated, then sat on the edge of his bed and looked at Joe. "You know…I'm falling for her in a big way."

"Hey, wait a minute. What about all the things you told me? Marriage and children weren't in your plans, you said. Not until there's a way to get rid of the HIV. All that made sense to me." Joe laid aside the surgical journal he'd been reading. "Giving the virus to a baby is not good for anybody, and you know that'd probably happen with Barbara positive and all."

"Yeah, I know. We talked about it. Barbara feels pretty much the same as I do about pregnancy. She may change my mind about getting married, though." He stretched out and folded a pillow beneath his head.

"Neither one of us is ready to commit to marriage yet, but we're talking about it."

"Damn, Jeremy, be careful. I like you both a lot. I'd sure hate to see either one of you get hurt."

"Thanks, Joe, I appreciate that." He sat up quickly. "And I like your idea about dinner tomorrow night. Let's do it."

Joe beamed. "Great. I'll take you to an Italian restaurant I discovered while you were gone. A place in the Quarter, a couple of blocks from the apartment." Turning back to the journal, he said, "I guess you heard we had another unexpected death."

"No. When?"

"While you were gone. A patient on my team, a woman with stage one breast cancer. Almost ready to go home, but she wanted to stay in the hospital an extra day to start testing for one of the HIV protocols." He began to doodle on a note pad. "It was the same as all the others. Sudden onset of fever, blood pressure bottomed out, then she became unconscious and died of progressive shock in about four hours' time."

"Exactly the same." Jeremy got up, went in the bathroom, and spoke over his shoulder while standing at the toilet. "My dad was impressed with the stuff you sent us—those chart reviews. He's talking about foul play, worried about some kind of conspiracy or something."

Joe looked at him sheepishly. "I know he's worried about it. He asked me to do those chart reviews."

"My dad asked you to do that?" Returning to the room, he stopped beside Joe's desk. "When, Joe? When did Dad ask you?"

"While he was here. I think it was that day you went to the HIV Lab."

Jeremy grinned. "Come on. You guys are ganging up on me. Was Barbara in on it, too?"

"No, she didn't even know about it. I told her it was my idea. Your father didn't want to worry either one of you."

"Well, he is a sly devil." He walked back to his bed. "Our senator's been a friend of my family for years. Dad called him and told him about all of it. The senator called back Monday morning—said he'd discovered something odd about the whole thing. He wouldn't say what it was, but he and Dad are supposed to get together in Beaumont this weekend to talk about it. He said we should keep the whole thing to ourselves for the time being."

Joe stood up from the desk. "Sounds serious. Can't we do anything? We're already in place. This is where it's all happening."

"Maybe…maybe we can do something, Joe." He hesitated.

"Barbara's not too happy about it, but there is one thing I want to check—"

The telephone rang, that hated klaxon that always interrupted one thing or another in the life of a surgery resident. Joe's junior resident needed him in the ICU. Then, before Joe returned, Jeremy was called to the Emergency Room to help his team take care of a young man who had been involved in an automobile crash.

❖ ❖ ❖

32

The Accident Victim

Jeremy reached the ER in the midst of the seemingly chaotic early treatment for major trauma. Orderly, not chaotic the way it looked, it was business as usual in a major trauma center. In Number One Trauma Room a crowd of doctors, nurses and medical students buzzed around a patient who was lying naked beneath a ceiling mounted spotlight.

The man's head was blood smeared and strapped tightly in position, allowing no movement in his potentially injured neck. Tubes and catheters emerged from every part of his body. Intravenous fluids dripped rapidly into each arm. His left leg was enclosed in an inflatable air splint, and a drainage tube entered his chest through a small incision on the left side of his rib cage. Acrid smells of human stress filled the small room. A bubbling suction device attached to the chest tube gave an oddly playful sound to the macabre scene.

As gruesome as it appeared, Jeremy knew every movement of each team member had a purpose. Each tube, each observation, played a very specific role in the breakneck drama of trying to counteract the patient's injuries and keep him alive. It was not the satanic ritual it appeared to be, but a carefully planned series of actions that gave the man his best chance to survive.

As soon as Jeremy entered the room the junior resident pulled him aside to describe the patient's injuries. "He was driving a small car. Crashed through the guard rail of an overpass on Jeff Davis Parkway. No other passengers. His car was totaled when it hit the ground, but the patient was stable when the EMS crew got him out. They put that splint on his leg and brought him in Code 3."

Jeremy nodded. "How's he doing now?"

"That's the problem. He was stable at first, then he started going downhill fast and we're not sure why. That's when we called you."

"Who is he?"

"I don't know. Admitting has his wallet. I saw an M-E-P card from the Research Lab. He told us his name's Bob. Bob Anderson, I think he said."

"What have you found?" Jeremy asked. "You say his car went through the guard rail?"

"That's right. The EMS techs found him wearing a seat belt. They said he was conscious. He complained of knee pain—that's why they put that splint on his leg. He told 'em he suddenly got dizzy and lost control of the car." The resident pointed to the patient's head. "He had lots of bleeding from those cuts on his forehead, but EMS didn't really think he had a serious injury. Neither did we at first."

Jeremy raised his eyebrows. "He looks pretty bad now. What's his blood pressure?"

"Ninety-two over seventy. Pulse one twenty-eight."

"Did you give him any blood?"

"Not yet. They're still working on the cross match. We gave him two units of plasma expander. That's the third and fourth liters of lactated Ringers running right now."

"I better have a look," Jeremy said. He walked to the patient's side and put a hand on his shoulder. "Bob, open your eyes. Listen to me—I'm Dr. Becker. Open your eyes."

The patient did not respond. His breathing was rapid, though not obstructed. The bedside monitor displayed regular heart rhythm. Fast, but regular.

Jeremy reached for an ophthalmoscope and turned on its light. Lifting the man's eyelids with his fingers, he flashed the light in one eye, then the other. His pupils were the same size, both fully dilated, no response to the light.

Leaning close, Jeremy peered through the instrument's lens at the patient's retinas, deep inside his eyes. Nothing to suggest bleeding within the skull, no sign of increased pressure.

He twisted the ophthalmoscope head off the instrument's handle, then replaced it with an otoscope and looked into each of the patient's ears. Canals clean, no blood. Both TMs normal. No sign of blood in the middle ears.

Using a rubber hammer, he tapped the tendons at the man's elbows and his unsplinted knee, then drug his fingernail along the bottom of each foot. All reflexes were sluggish, otherwise normal and symmetrical.

Jeremy ran his fingers through the man's blood-caked hair, feeling for scalp wounds. No swelling, no lacerations. The blood must have come from his facial wounds.

He turned to the scrub sink and washed his hands, then pulled a stethoscope from his coat pocket and stretched its ear pieces around his neck. Before listening to the man's heart and lungs, he pressed both hands gently against his chest. Breathing symmetrical, no stridor. Damn, his skin was hot. "What's his temperature?"

The intern looked at the vital signs clipboard. "It was normal when he came in. We haven't taken it since then."

"Better check it again," Jeremy said. "Feel that skin."

The intern touched the patient and recoiled. "My god—he's hot as a firecracker." He looked at Jeremy with a puzzled expression. "Why would he have fever? He was injured less than two hours ago."

"You're right—it is odd," Jeremy glanced at the nurse. "Ask the admitting clerk to come over here while we take another temp. Maybe they've found out more about this guy." He turned to the junior resident. "Are you sure he was healthy before the wreck?"

"He told the ambulance crew he was. HIV-positive, but otherwise well."

"Have you found anything else? What about his aorta?" Jeremy knew a hidden tear in the wall of that huge artery in the chest could lead to progressive hemorrhage and death.

"We thought about that, but his chest x-ray looks okay and his leg pulses are normal. He did have a pneumothorax. We thought that might've caused his shock, but he didn't improve after we put the chest tube in."

Jeremy looked at the x-rays of the man's chest and head on the lighted view box. "Other than about fifty percent pneumothorax and this rib fracture, the films look okay to me. What do you think?"

"I agree," the resident said. "We tapped his pericardium and did abdominal lavage. Both normal. We were ready to take him for a CAT scan when he started to fall apart."

"Blood gases?"

"No problem there, all normal."

A new face appeared at the door, an efficient looking young woman with smooth café-au-lait skin peeked in. "You wanted to see me, Dr. Becker? I'm from Admitting."

Jeremy glanced around the room to be sure the others were doing everything needed for the patient, then nodded to the admitting clerk and joined her in the hall. "What have you found out about this patient—Anderson is he?"

The clerk glanced at the worksheet on her clipboard. "That's right, Robert Anderson. He works across the street at the HIV Lab. His next of kin is in Connecticut, so I called the duty officer at the Lab. They verified his ID number. Said they'd notify his supervisor. We oughta hear more from 'em soon. It's been about forty minutes."

"Anything else? Any kind of medical ID?"

She ran a slender finger down the worksheet. "We read the medical info from his HIV card. No major illnesses, no surgery, blood type O positive."

"Any idea where he works at the Research Lab?"

"Let's see...here it is. He works in Viro…something."

"Virology?"

"That's right—that's what the duty officer said, the Virology Section."

"Okay, thanks. Let me know if you learn anything new." Jeremy returned to the Trauma Room.

The intern said, "His temp's 103.6, Jeremy. We're trying to cool him down. Should I take him for the CAT scan?"

"Forget it, he's too unstable right now."

The coffee-skinned clerk poked her head through the door again. "Dr. Becker?"

He looked at her and raised his eyebrows.

"Mr. Anderson's supervisor is here. Can you talk to him?"

Jeremy nodded, then turned to the junior resident. "Try to get his temp down. Can you think of anything else?"

"Not a thing."

Jeremy stepped back through the door and looked around. The clerk was standing just down the hall talking to a tall, lanky man wearing a tweed sport jacket and jeans. Damn, it was Daniel Hebert from the HIV Lab—Jeremy headed in their direction.

"Jeremy," Hebert said. "I'm glad to see you're here. How is Anderson? Does he have a serious injury?"

"Anderson's not doing too well, Dan. I forgot he'd be from your section. Do you know anything about his medical background?"

"Nothing significant that I know about, nothing other than HIV-positive. I called his family—they're making arrangements to come down here. His father didn't mention any health problems. I can call them back if you want me to ask anything special."

"No, that's okay. We'll just—"

The nurse opened the door of the trauma room. "Dr. Becker, you'd better come in."

Jeremy realized at a glance the injured patient's condition was worse. Even as he watched, the EKG monitor changed from a rapid regular heart rhythm to the erratic, ineffective twitching of ventricular fibrillation. He and the others treated the lethal heart rhythm aggressively, but nothing changed it. In three quarters of an hour the man was dead.

Jeremy found Daniel Hebert in a waiting room just outside the main treatment area. He was standing at a desk, speaking on the telephone, his back toward the door. Waiting, Jeremy could not avoid overhearing Hebert say, "That's right, Bob Anderson from the NOLA lab. The doctors say he's not doing well."

Hebert listened for a moment. "Of course, they're doing everything." He listened again, then became agitated. "No, Marshall, you don't need to come over here."

Hebert looked up and saw Jeremy. "I have to go now—the doctor's here." He hung up without waiting for a response. "How's Bob? His family can get a plane out of New Haven in about an hour."

"Dan, I'm sorry to tell you this, but Anderson is dead."

"Dead? My God, I didn't think he was hurt that bad." Hebert paled visibly and sat down.

"He probably didn't die of his injuries," Jeremy said. "It's pretty strange, actually. He responded like a patient with an uncontrollable infection and progressive septic shock. Can you tell me anything more about him?"

Hebert shook his head. "Nothing. You know he worked in the Virology Section. He was assigned to our lab that looks after the cultures of the NOLA strain."

"The HIV-NOLA strain?"

"That's right." Hebert grimaced and his shoulders slumped. He got up and walked to the window. "There was an minor accident in that lab this afternoon. Anderson cut his hand on a broken pipette. It was—he said it was—a clean, unused pipette. It was a small cut, so we didn't send him to the medical section. Could that have anything to do with Anderson's auto accident?"

Jeremy shook his head. "I doubt it. Maybe the autopsy'll answer that question."

"Autopsy? Who'll authorize an autopsy?"

"The coroner will require one. He'll order it because of the Anderson's death following an injury."

"Is that routine?"

"Yes, it's a legal requirement."

Ignoring Hebert's skeptical look, Jeremy said, "Will you telephone his family again? I'll be glad to talk to them later, but at the moment you can tell them everything I could."

"Sure, I can do that." Hebert raised his eyebrows. "May I tell 'em you'll give me a report of the autopsy?"

Puzzled, Jeremy looked at him.

Hebert shrugged and said, "So I can pass it along to the family."

"Oh. Okay...sure. Tell 'em it'll be two or three weeks before we have anything to report."

Leaving Hebert, Jeremy returned to the trauma room. One more thing to check on while the staff prepared the body for removal to the morgue. He looked at Anderson's hands, and there it was. In the web space between his right thumb and index finger. A fresh cut. Small. Didn't look deep. No sign of infection—unlikely that such a trivial injury could have anything to do with Anderson's unexpected death.

Early the following morning, Jeremy showed up at the coroner's autopsy on Bob Anderson. He wanted to discover whether he and his team had failed to recognize some lethal injury. He needed to understand why their patient's lack of response had suggested infection and not trauma.

As soon as he entered the morgue's outer door he ran into an overwhelming chemical odor. Oil of wintergreen. The deaners who clean morgues probably all learn to use that stuff to cover up more obnoxious smells. It always made Jeremy think of some weird kind of candy store.

This morgue's deaner was an aged black man who performed his chores with skill and great dignity. When Jeremy walked in, the old man looked up and nodded his head of curly white hair. He had stretched Anderson's naked body out on the perforated surface of a dissecting table, a table with a lower chamber to drain liquids away during the autopsy. Instruments that looked like a grotesque combination of operating room and butcher shop were arranged nearby in neat rows.

Jeremy recognized the pathology resident seated at a counter on one side of the room, poring over the patient's hospital chart. "Good morning, Dr. Sweet. Will you be doing this autopsy?"

The pathologist was a short man with thinning hair and dark complexion. He turned and peered over the top of his tortoise shell glasses. "What? Oh, hello, Jeremy. Sure, I'll be doing the post. The coroner released it to us." Dr. Sweet stood up and walked toward the dissecting table. "I see your team took care of him. Why do you think he died?"

"I really don't know, Mike. We didn't find any lethal injury. He responded more like septic shock."

Sweet adjusted his glasses and pulled on a pair of rubber gloves. "Yeah, the chart does sound like sepsis all right. I collected a sterile blood sample from his heart for cultures."

"Virus cultures, I hope."

"Right, I put some of it in virus medium." He turned toward the body, then looked at the deaner. "Well, let's find out. All set, Rudy?"

"All set, doctor." Rudy sprayed the dead man's entire body with clear water to make it easier to clean when the autopsy was finished. He opened a specimen bottle containing formaldehyde, and that new stink overpowered the oil of wintergreen.

Sweet picked up a large bladed scalpel and made a long Y-shaped incision that extended across Anderson's chest and abdomen, from his shoulders to his pubis. While Jeremy watched, he examined every internal organ, collecting a small sample of each for microscopic study.

Jeremy opened an instrument pack containing a sterile scalpel. He pulled on a pair of sterile gloves and collected bits of the deep tissues from the wound on the man's right hand for virus cultures. He reminded Dr. Sweet to sample his spleen and lungs for virus cultures as well.

"Everything looks normal so far," Sweet said. "We'd better have a look at the brain."

Using a concealed incision from ear to ear beneath the man's hair, Rudy peeled back his scalp and opened the skull with an electric saw. Dr. Sweet's meticulous examination of the virologist's skull and his brain disclosed no abnormality. The autopsy did not demonstrate a cause for his death.

Jeremy was relieved to find no unexpected injuries, but they'd also failed to find an explanation for Anderson's rapid deterioration. He knew the virus cultures would take several weeks, and the microscopic studies of his organs were not likely to come up with anything new.

They had reached an impasse. The final answers to the team's questions would have to wait, and Jeremy could do nothing more. Nothing but wait and wonder why this accident victim's death had been so much like the other deaths they'd seen in hospital patients. It made no sense, none at all.

❖❖❖

33

JOE'S STORY

IN THE EARLY EVENING, HALF AN HOUR LATER THAN HE HAD hoped, Jeremy hurried through the courtyard of the Burgundy Street apartment. He got hung up at the hospital, and he knew Joe was counting on the dinner plans they'd made. Certain Joe was already at the apartment, he didn't bother with a key, didn't even knock. He just pushed the door open and spotted Joe leaning over the dresser, close to the mirror. Wearing only a towel wrapped around his waist, he was pressing his fingers against the side of his neck, like he was giving himself a physical.

Joe yelled and jumped back from the mirror. "Jesus, you scared the shit out of me."

"Sorry," Jeremy laughed. "I should've knocked or something."

Joe shrugged. "It's all right. I'm always a little jumpy when I'm alone in this place. I must've forgotten to lock the door." He waved toward the reflection of his towel clad body. "I just got out of the shower. Give me a minute to get dressed."

"Take your time. This is our night off, remember?"

Joe tossed the towel aside and stepped into a pair of bright yellow bikini briefs.

"Are you losing weight?" Jeremy asked. "You look thin."

Joe patted himself on the belly. "Maybe a little." He turned sideways and looked in the mirror. "I've always burned it off faster than I put it on. Papa used to tell me it was the Italian blood."

Jeremy smiled. "You look thinner than usual to me. Better keep an eye on it." He handed Joe the shirt he'd hung over the back of a chair and grinned. "I know what's wrong with you—you need a good Italian dinner."

"Right." Joe beamed. "Wait 'til you see this place. The owner's really happy to find somebody who speaks a little Italian. I called and asked him to make us a special dinner."

"Great." Jeremy picked up a baseball bat and glove from the floor beside the dresser and put them away on the closet shelf. "Sorry about leaving this stuff laying around. Not much of a housekeeper, am I?"

"Don't worry about it—doesn't bother me."

Jeremy glanced at his watch. "How about a drink on the patio before we go? I'd like to tell you about a patient we lost in the ER last night."

The still, hot evenings of summer in the Vieux Carré had given way to early autumn, and the courtyard was especially inviting despite the ever-present humidity. They sat near the fountain with their drinks, and Jeremy described his team's frustrating treatment of the injured virologist.

Joe agreed the man's death probably wasn't caused by the auto accident. "It sounds a lot like our hospital deaths, doesn't it?" He sipped his drink. Cold condensate from the glass dripped on his thigh and he blotted it with a napkin. "You think it could have been something infectious—something that's spread to the ER?"

"I don't know what the hell it is," Jeremy said. "But it worries me." He put his glass on the table and lowered his voice. "There's another thing I want to talk to you about—that business about lab techs drawing blood from the patients who died on the wards. I still think that's related, somehow, to their deaths."

Joe shook his head. "You never let go of that idea do you? We talked about it when your dad was here, remember? Didn't the Chief satisfy you with whatever he found out?"

"Not really. I thought about it a lot while I was in Beaumont." He paused a half beat. "I want you to help me check it out."

Joe hesitated. "What do you mean, check it out? What can we do?"

Jeremy got up from his chair. "Hey, you're the one who asked if we couldn't do something while we're waiting to hear from Senator Randall. This may be it." He paced silently for a moment. "I don't know whether the lab drew blood from all the patients, but I think we could use your chart reviews to find out. Identify the nurses who were on duty when each patient died. Talk to the nurses, see if they remember who drew the blood."

Joe frowned and scratched his head. "I guess we could do that, but I doubt…." Suddenly he looked up. "What about your patient in the ER? Did a lab tech come down there?"

"Good question. I don't think anybody from the lab was there." Jeremy hesitated, then rushed on. "I'm sure no lab tech drew blood after I got to the ER. I'll have to ask the others what happened before they called me." He stopped pacing and sat down. "But there is something else, Joe—another thing that might relate to the hospital deaths."

"What do you mean?"

Jeremy stabbed a finger toward Joe. "You discovered all of the patients were volunteers for one of the HIV protocols, remember?" He waited for Joe to nod in agreement. "My patient in the ER was a virologist at the Research Facility. Could the HIV Lab be the common denominator?"

Joe shook his head. "I don't think so. None of the ward patients had actually started a treatment protocol. They'd just had a few preliminary tests to qualify for the clinical trials—the research lab wasn't really involved with any of them. That's probably a coincidence anyway. A lot of our patients volunteer for the HIV protocols, and not many of 'em die."

"Yeah, I guess you're right."

"How about this idea?" Joe said. "All the hospital patients were HIV positive, right? Your accident victim must have been positive, too. Could it be some new mutation of the virus?"

"Maybe…Anderson was HIV-positive. We had his M-E-P card." He smiled at Joe. "I've gotten so used to all our patients being positive, I didn't even think about it while we were working on him." But Joe's question raised a frightening possibility. "God, I hope you're wrong about a new mutation—we're positive, too, remember?"

"I wish I could forget it." Joe lifted his glass and downed the last of his drink. "I've never told you about my own HIV conversion, have I?"

"No, I don't think you have, but it's not important."

Joe looked directly at his roommate. "It's important to me, Jeremy." He touched the side of his neck with his fingertips. "I know about your accident with that patient in med school. I want to tell you how it happened to me."

Jeremy freshened their drinks, and Joe began his story, speaking slowly and deliberately. His face made it clear that some of his recollections were painful.

"I was about ten years old when Francisco Maggiano became my father's apprentice in the deli. Frank, that's what we called him, Frank was fifteen at the time." He glanced at Jeremy and raised his eyebrows, then settled into a story-telling voice. "He'd just come to the States, you know? His father and Papa were boyhood friends. Grew up in the same village. Frank learned the business quickly, and pretty soon he was more of a partner than an apprentice. He lived with us and, in many ways, he was like an older brother to me."

"Joe—"

He waved off Jeremy's interruption. "Papa opened his bar about that time. You know how much he likes that bar. His prize winning *Pousse-café* and all that stuff."

Jeremy nodded.

"On weekends and during the summer when school was out, I took over Frank's job in the deli so he could start working with Papa in the bar. I would have done just about anything to help Frank." He fell silent for a moment, then smiled. "I worked my tail off to run the deli the same way Frank had. To please Papa, you know, so Frank could learn the bar business."

"Joe, this sounds like pretty personal stuff. You don't have to tell me about it."

"I know I don't, Jeremy, but I want to." He grew thoughtful as he slipped back into his boyhood. "After a year or two, when Frank was comfortable with English, he began to spend his free time away from the family. By the time I was fifteen, I knew most of Frank's friends were gay and I was angry about that—jealous I guess, though I didn't realize it at the time. Frank was a beautiful person. I idolized him. I wanted to be a part of his life. I told him I didn't like some of his friends, but he said, 'Don't worry about it, Little Joe.' He liked to call me Little Joe. He said, 'I'm gay because I want to be. That's the way I like it. But I can still be with you.'"

"I've heard you mention Frank," Jeremy said, "but I didn't know you were so close."

"I was closer to Frank than any of my real brothers." A lot closer...." Joe smiled again and looked up at the evening sky. "Gradually—over the next two or three years—he introduced me to homosexuality. I knew exactly what I was doing. I was eager to express my love for that man openly, physically."

The story was beginning to be more than Jeremy had bargained for. He finished his drink and waited for the ending.

"Frank and I had an on-again, off-again affair for about eight years. None of the family knew about it, of course. In the third year of med school, the first time they tested us for HIV, my test was positive." He paused and shook his head. "That devastated Papa. His son, the doctor, had the queers' disease. It was the beginning of my isolation from the family.

"Since then I've lived for the hope of a cure before I develop AIDS." Joe took a swallow of his drink, then put the glass down and tugged at his collar. "That new treatment plan sounds good, but you know we can't use it until the clinical safety trials are finished. And you're supposed to be in charge of enrolling patients for the trials. Hell, you're gonna be so busy checking out this other stuff—" His voice cracked. "Why can't we just forget about the patient deaths? Let your senator check that out. Let's get moving on the protocols. God, Jeremy, we may be running out of time. I don't want to die of AIDS."

Jeremy walked over and put his hand on Joe's shoulder. "We've got enough time. I'm ready to sign up volunteers for the safety trials right now. Checking out the deaths won't take time away from that."

Joe looked away and his hand went to his neck again.

"What became of Frank?" Jeremy asked. "Where is he now?"

"Still in New Orleans, I think. He drifted away from my family after I tested positive. He had to be positive, too, but he didn't tell us the results of his blood test. Papa told the rest of us Frank left to go in business for himself, but I found out he was living in the Garden District—living with an older man. I saw them together in the bars once or twice, but I haven't seen Frank since then. A bartender told me the other man died of AIDS a couple of years ago, but I haven't heard a single word from Frank."

After a long silence Jeremy said, "I don't know what to say, Joe."

Looking relieved, Joe got up and cleared their empty glasses from the table. "You don't have to say anything. I needed to talk about it, that's all. Thanks for listening." He grinned. "Enough of that stuff. Let's go get some dinner. I guarantee we're going to a real Italian kitchen tonight."

The owner and chef of the tiny restaurant on Ursulines Street personally welcomed his paisano, *il dottore*. Joe called him Raphael. He was a short, round-faced man who looked like food was an important part of his life. He shook Jeremy's hand, then pulled him into a bear hug like the one he'd given Joe. "*Buona sera! Benvenuto! Piacere!* Good evening. Welcome. Pleased to meet you." Rich smells of sautéing garlic and onions swirled around him.

Raphael seated them at a candle-lit table in the center of the small dining room, then brought a chilled bottle of white Montevecchio, which Jeremy learned was rarely seen outside the Lombardy district where it's grapes grew. Raphael told them this bottle was from a single case he had somehow obtained from relatives in Como. It suited the *antipasti*, a huge plate of appetizers with a stuffed artichoke as its centerpiece. The stuffing was a garlic lover's delight.

"I could make a meal of that artichoke," Jeremy said. "When do we get to see the menu?"

"No menu tonight. I don't even know what we're having—Raphael planned it all."

"It'll cost a fortune, Joe. That rare wine and everything. Just so there's no misunderstanding, we're splitting this check."

Joe smiled. "Okay. But don't be surprised if there is no check. I'm pretty sure this is Raphael's treat."

Before Jeremy could protest, the main course arrived, *vitello saltimbocca* surrounded by a medley of fresh garden vegetables. Raphael brought a red Bardolino which he had opened earlier, and a generous side dish of pasta in marinara sauce. He poured a small glass of the wine for himself and toasted his guests, then waited for them to taste the veal. It really did melt in your mouth, Jeremy discovered. "Man, this veal's got to be as good as any *saltimbocca* prepared in Milano."

As soon as they finished that course, the table was cleared and Raphael presented a plate of salad greens dressed with extra virgin olive oil and a splash of balsamic from Modena. He said something to Joe in Italian.

"He needs a few minutes to fix our dessert," Joe explained. "We should take our time with the salad."

"There's more coming? Raphael's incredible. He could have the best restaurant in town."

"He doesn't want a bigger place," Joe said. "Everybody working here is family—he wants to keep it that way."

"I'm glad he likes you. What did you do? Offer him free surgery for the rest of his life?"

Joe grinned. "You just have to speak the right language."

A young woman placed dessert dishes in front of them, then signaled toward the kitchen door. Raphael appeared, still whipping the contents of a steaming sauce pan with a wire whisk. He rushed to the table and stirred a creamy, beige custard into their dishes. *Zabaglione*, a hot egg custard made with Marsala wine.

The server brought cups of *espresso* and a plate of sweet *biscotti*. Jeremy caught the rich, fragrance of Marsala rising from the hot custard, as Raphael explained that *zabaglione* needed to sprint, *presto*, from the fire to the mouth. After one taste, Joe made grateful comments in Italian which must have been complimentary because Raphael just stood there, beaming. Sensuous people, Jeremy thought. These Italians.

Dinner finished, they declined the server's offer of *grappa*, and Joe went to the kitchen to talk to Raphael about the check. They returned together, and Raphael escorted Joe and Jeremy to the door with a flurry of gestures and a noisy, bilingual discussion about when they might return. There was no check. When they reached the sidewalk Joe stopped and smiled at Jeremy. "*Molto bene, no?* Very nice, huh?"

"*Si,*" Jeremy said, grinning. "*Bellisimo!*"

34

An Odd Couple

Jeremy noticed Joe's mood had improved steadily during their evening out. He seemed elated by the success of their dinner, and Jeremy was not really surprised when he suggested drinks at a bar on the way back to the apartment.

"I'm not much for bars," Jeremy said. "But I could go for something light. Where do you want to go?"

"I was thinking of a place over on Governor Nicholls Street called The Eagle—I know a couple of guys who work there."

"The Eagle? Isn't that a gay bar?"

"Well, yes...but you don't have to be gay to go there. There are lots—"

"I don't know, Joe. I wouldn't know what to do in a place like that."

"Do? You don't need to do anything. Just have a drink. Aside from the sexual preference of most of the patrons, it's not much different from any other bar."

Jeremy raised his eyebrows. "That's not what I've heard."

Joe laughed out loud. "I don't know what you've heard, but this is a pretty nice place." Then, smiling, he punched Jeremy's shoulder. "If anybody makes a pass, just tell 'em you're with me."

Caught up in the humor of the situation, Jeremy laughed. He didn't feel threatened by the idea of going to a gay bar. No use to make a big deal out of it. Joe had been so depressed earlier—no harm in helping him stay up. "Okay, buddy. I don't know exactly why, but you're on. Let's go."

The Eagle was a short walk away, on a street corner. The tall double doors of its entry were cut diagonally across the corner of the building. The M-E-P was skillfully decorated with wrought iron to make it as unobtrusive as possible. They entered a dimly lighted room more than half filled by a dark, U-shaped wooden bar with a gleaming brass foot rail. The place reeked of beer and cigarette smoke and old wood. Plaintive sounds of country music floated through the smoky air from ceiling-mounted speakers.

Every head at the crowded bar swiveled toward Joe and Jeremy when they walked through the door. Despite the dim light, Jeremy could see they were all men—men who, for the most part, would not have appeared out of place in any social gathering.

Looking for seats they headed toward the bar, moving slowly in the dark room. A strapping blond seated at a barstool looked up. Fortyish, with tightly curled, sheep-like hair, he turned on his stool and clapped a muscular arm around Joe's shoulders. "Joe-Joe, how're you doing? Long time no see. Where've you been?

"Hey, Carl. I'm fine." He smiled. "It has been a while, hasn't it? Working too hard, I guess." He turned to withdraw from the man's half-embrace and pulled Jeremy into the conversation. "Carl, this is my friend, Jeremy Becker. Carl Delahousay."

Jeremy took the hand extended toward him. "Hello, Carl. Good to meet you."

Carl wore a smooth fitting tee shirt emblazoned with The Eagle's logo beneath a soaring bird of prey. His firm handshake matched his physique. "Thanks," he said. "Always glad to meet a friend of Joe's." He beamed at Joe, flashing perfectly aligned teeth, then pointed toward two empty seats at one end of the bar, then at the bartender . "Why don't you guys sit over there. Tell Lyle what you want to drink. It's on me."

"Thanks," Joe said. "Thanks a lot."

Carl winked at Jeremy. "It's my pleasure." He stretched out his hand for another shake. This time Jeremy noticed Carl's palm was hard with calluses.

Joe led the way toward the empty barstools, greeting several other men as they passed through the crowd. Some of them wore sport jackets with open shirts or ties loosened at the neck—others jeans and tee shirts. Most of the jeans looked worn or faded, all of them crotch huggers. Tightest jeans Jeremy'd ever seen.

Lyle, the bartender, wore a shirt like Carl's, though not as well filled by his slender young body. He served their drinks, and Jeremy saw Carl raise a toast when he picked up his own glass. He smiled broadly and returned the gesture as he leaned toward Joe. "Where's the john? I'm about to pop."

"Right over there, on the other side of the pool table." He stopped Jeremy with a look. "But I don't think you should go right now."

"Why not? I've waited about as long as I can."

"You'd better wait a few more minutes."

"Why should I wait? What's going on?"

"More than you think." Joe stifled a laugh. "Old Carl's making a play for you."

"What? You're crazy." He shook his head. "I told you I wouldn't know what to do in this place."

"That's the problem. You're doing too much."

"What're you talking about? I haven't done a thing."

"It's very subtle, Jeremy. You're not used to it." He tapped his head with his fingers. "After a while you develop a little sensor that signals when somebody's cruising—we call it gaydar. You learn how to respond."

Jeremy shrugged and put his glass down. "Okay, whatever you say. But what did I do wrong?"

"Nothing wrong, but I'm afraid Carl thinks you're interested."

"What? How could he—"

"It's the way you smiled when you returned his toast. A little too friendly. If you go to the can right now, he'll probably follow you. He'll think it's a signal from you."

"This is too complicated for me, Joe. I'd better get out of here."

"You don't have to leave. Enjoy your drink. Just try not to look at Carl for a while. And wait a few minutes before you go to the men's room."

Jeremy was careful to keep his gaze straight ahead. A rectangular lamp of fake stained glass hung low over a green felt pool table, creating an island of light in the dark room. One of the players, a young man wearing jeans, looked like an everyday, clean-cut junior executive. Clean-cut except for his garb. He wore a tight fitting leather vest, but he was otherwise bare from the waist up.

The other player.... Could it be? Yes, an attractive young woman in jeans and a western shirt. Jeremy watched as she put her cigarette on the edge of the table and took a bead on the cue ball. Shrieks of delight rose over the music when she sank the thirteen with an impossible-looking two cushion shot. It was the last stripe on the table, and her opponent looked dejected as she lined up the eight ball for an easy straight-in shot.

The man in the leather vest shook his head and winked at the girl as he mouthed, "Women!" He dug in the pocket of his tight jeans and slapped two quarters on the edge of the table.

Lyle, the bartender, came over, wiping the bar with a towel. "Another round?

Joe declined and turned to Jeremy. "I think it's safe for you to go to the men's room now. Carl's found a friend."

"Who is Carl anyway?" Jeremy asked.

Lyle leaned close to them and said, "Carl's a piranha."

Jeremy was baffled. Even Joe raised his eyebrows. "What?"

"A piranha," Lyle said. "He's a sexual piranha in an age when carnivores are out of fashion."

Jeremy and Joe both laughed. Joe said, "Carl owns a building company—Delahousay Renovations."

"That's Delahousay? I see his signs all over town."

Joe smiled. "That's him. Pretty big outfit."

"Really," Jeremy said.

"I told you this was a nice place. You never know who'll be here." He looked around the room and tilted his head toward the man in the vest. "See that guy playing pool?"

Jeremy nodded.

"He's an attorney from the DA's office. Promising career, I hear."

Jeremy realized how little he knew about most of the people in The Eagle. Freud was right. Every one of them wore alter egos like costumes to disguise their workaday identities. Which one's the disguise? he wondered. Which one real? He swiveled his stool toward Joe and stood up. "I'm going to the john now," he said. "If you order another drink I'll have one, too."

"Okay. Brandy-soda?"

"Right—lemon twist."

Jeremy moved through the crowd in the direction Joe had indicated. When he passed the pool table, the leather-vested attorney gave him an unmistakable once over, then an inviting smile. Without thinking, he returned the smile. Oh, shit! Better watch that.

Turning into an anteroom which he expected to lead to the restrooms, he found the walls covered with posters of incredibly endowed muscle beach types in various stages of undress. A vending machine for condoms was featured prominently among them, and there were two doors, labeled "Men" and "Ladies". So far, so good. His confidence grew.

A distinguished looking man walked out of the "Ladies", checking his fly in a way that made it clear why he'd been inside. He noticed Jeremy's surprise and smiled. "There're never enough ladies here to have a room of their own, so I use it for 'em." He jabbed his thumb toward the Men's. "A lot more private than that place."

At that moment, a woman came through the "Men's" door—at least

Jeremy thought it was a woman, until he noticed her large Adam's apple and tufts of chest hair sprouting above her low cut gown. She spoke to him in a masculine voice. "Hello, darling. Where've you been all my life?"

Confused now, he looked around and spotted a group of men at the top of the stairs rising from the opposite side of the anteroom. Maybe there was a regular men's room up there. He went up and was surprised to find another bar. Several men were standing around, talking to a burly bartender dressed in a sleeveless buckskin shirt, jeans, and cowboy boots.

The country music was louder upstairs. A dance floor filled about half of the room, and Jeremy was astonished to see several couples, all men, gliding round and round in a smooth Texas two-step. Damn, he thought. Knowing about this stuff's one thing—seeing it's something else. The men danced together with a grace he'd never imagined. Faces expressionless, each couple spinning in perfect tempo with the music, like porcelain figures on a Victorian music box.

"Hi, good looking. How'd you like to trip the light fantastic?" The deep voice startled Jeremy and he whirled around to find he was looking directly at a man's bare chest. The guy had to be nearly seven feet tall. He wore jeans and western boots with leather chaps, but no shirt.

"Didn't mean to spook you," the giant said. He smiled and held out his hand. "My name's Sam. Would you like to dance?"

"What? No. No thank you, Sam."

"Hey, you sound like you might be from Texas. What's your name?"

"Jeremy. I'm from Beaumont."

"Well, I'll be." He grabbed Jeremy's hand and gave it a vigorous shake. "I'm from Abilene, myself. Who'd believe it—finding another Texas boy, smack dab in the middle of the French Quarter."

"Uh, Sam, I'm looking for the men's room. Do you know where it is?"

"Sure do." He pointed to the opposite side of the room. "Right over there by those steps going up to the third floor. Go on in there and hurry back." He grinned. "Unless you want me to help you."

Jeremy shook his head. "No thanks, I can manage." He was afraid to smile.

Big Sam grabbed him by the arm and lowered his voice. "Don't waste your time going up the stairs. Nothing up there but a bunch of kids and all that disco stuff. The good dancin's down here. I'll get you a beer while you pee."

"No, thanks, Sam. I left a drink downstairs with my friend." The giant looked crestfallen. Jeremy made his way to the restroom and gratefully closed the door behind him. To his chagrin, the room was not empty.

The urinal was a long trough filled to the brim with crushed ice. Three men stood there with their backs to Jeremy, evenly spaced along the trough. The primitive bass beat of the third floor disco pounded through the ceiling of the dingy room. Generations of users had covered the walls with graffiti that shouted the clarion call of their rage, their loneliness. The man at the center of the urinal stepped away, rearranging himself in his jeans.

Ignoring him, Jeremy stepped up to the trough, taking the vacant spot. He noticed a mirror above the urinal was tilted slightly downward, then he saw why. There was no way to keep from seeing exactly what everybody else at the trough was doing. Too late to back out now—he was fully committed to the task at hand when he noticed the man on his left. He was standing there—just standing, equipment in hand. Not urinating, just holding his enormous penis. He'd unbuttoned his western shirt to expose a tight body underneath.

In the mirror Jeremy saw the man's glassy eyes were staring directly at him. His bladder froze in mid-stream. He was in the wrong place for sure. He zipped his fly and left the restroom at full speed. He hesitated at the door just long enough to be sure Big Sam wouldn't see him, then bolted down the stairs to the main lounge. Slowing to a casual walk, he glanced to the left, to the far side of the pool table, and the biggest surprise of the evening stopped him dead in his tracks.

He recognized the two men sitting at a small table in a dark corner behind the pool table, practically under the stairs. He couldn't hear them, but their gestures betrayed angry words passing back and forth between them. As he watched, one of them stood up, longneck beer in hand, and leaned across the table to shake his fist in the other's face. Jesus, Jeremy thought. He couldn't believe it. He damn sure hoped those two hadn't seen him.

Jeremy waited, out of sight he hoped, until a crowd around the pool table blocked the view from the dark corner, then he headed back to the bar where Joe was sitting.

Joe turned from the man he'd been talking to and pushed a drink across the bar toward Jeremy. "Hey, guy, where've you been? I was about ready to send out a search party." He looked at the glass and wrinkled his nose. "You may not want this. The ice's probably melted."

"It doesn't matter. I don't want another drink anyway. Let's get out of here."

"Hold on, Jeremy. What's wrong? Are you okay?" He looked toward the restrooms. "What happened in there?"

"I'm fine." Jeremy leaned to look around the crowd. "Leonard Guidry's in this place. Right over there behind the pool table."

"Who's Leonard Guidry?" Joe shook his head slowly. "Hey listen, it doesn't matter who sees you in a gay bar. Don't forget, they're here, too."

"That's not the problem. Guidry's a housekeeper at the hospital. You must've seen him around the wards."

"Oh yeah, Cajun Lennie. But I still don't understand...."

One hand on the bar, Jeremy pointed toward the dark corner. "Guidry's sitting over there in the corner with Daniel Hebert from the virology lab. Those two are an unlikely couple if I ever saw one".

"You're making too much of it," Joe said. "You'll see lots of odd couples in a place like this."

"It's not that. They're having a pretty hot discussion back there—almost going at each other's throats." He thought about the surprising pair for a minute—remembered Guidry's visit to the infirmary and Hebert's tour of the HIV Lab. "I don't like it, Joe. I don't know what's going on with those two, but let's get out of here before they see us."

"I told you—don't worry about who sees us." Joe started to laugh, but Jeremy shot him a look that stopped him short. Levity gone, Joe asked, "What do you think it means, those guys being here? Why are you so upset about it?"

"I don't know exactly why—just a feeling I have. There's no reason for them to even know each other." He shook his head. "Another thing—one or the other of those two keeps popping up around the hospital. They've gotta be more than just some odd couple."

Joe looked puzzled. "What do you mean? You think maybe they had something to do with the patient deaths?"

Jeremy whirled toward him, vague thoughts meshing together with sudden clarity. "Yes, that's it. That's exactly what I think. I believe they're deliberately meeting in a gay bar so nobody'll notice 'em. And if I'm right, I sure as hell don't want 'em to know we saw them."

Joe peered through the crowd to get a look at the suspicious pair. "Didn't you tell me Dr. Hebert's from south Louisiana—same as Cajun Lennie?" He raised his eyebrows several times and mimicked puffing on a large cigar like Groucho Marx. "Maybe they're old buddies from the bayou. Meeting in a gay bar for Auld Lang Syne."

"Don't make a joke out of it. I'm serious. Come on—I'm out of here. Either one of those guys would know me in a minute. Guidry'd probably recognize you, Joe. Let's go."

35

Dr. Hollander

For nearly an hour after leaving The Eagle, Jeremy and Joe talked, sometimes argued, about why Leonard Guidry and Daniel Hebert were together in the bar. What in God's name was that unlikely couple up to? A housekeeper and a PhD virologist? What were they quarreling about? Did it have anything to do with the hospital—or was just a lovers' quarrel and nothing more?

They never agreed upon a logical explanation for the unexpected meeting they'd stumbled upon, not even when they picked up the discussion again the following morning at breakfast. They never figured it out, but something about it sounded dangerous to them—too dangerous to ignore. "We need to keep an eye on both of those guys," Jeremy said, "but I don't know how to do it."

Joe held up his hands. "Hold on, Jere. We're getting way too involved here. We're not in the detective business."

"Do you have a better idea?"

"Maybe we should go to the police."

Jeremy shook his head. "I don't think so. Not yet. We're not even sure they're doing anything wrong—the police'd probably just laugh at us."

"What about a private investigator?"

"That's a pretty good idea, but we'd play hell sneaking a private eye into Charity. I hear they're pretty expensive anyway."

Joe said, "Yeah, I guess you're right. We'll have to do it ourselves."

"That's what I think. We can't wait around either. I believe more of our patients are in danger—shit, we may even be in danger ourselves."

Joe took a swallow of coffee. "Why would those two want to mess with our patients?"

"I don't know why, Joe." Jeremy was getting impatient. "But that's damn sure what we need to find out.

"What about your senator?"

"Joe, we can't wait for Senator Randall. He can figure out the political angles, but this is a hospital problem. If our patients are in danger, we can't wait for a bunch of federal bureaucrats to plod through the whole thing."

"We can't do much without help. We have to get somebody else involved—we need to talk to the administrator or somebody."

Jeremy remembered his father's admonition. "Not a bad idea, but we'll have to talk to somebody besides Mr. Lockhart. Dad's already involved in this thing—you know how he feels about Lockhart."

Joe chuckled. "Yeah, I remember." He was silent for a while, then pushed his breakfast tray away and sat up straight. "I've got it. Let's talk to Dr. Hollander. Education's pretty involved with the front office, but Hollander's not like those other admin types. He'll listen to us—we can talk to him."

Jeremy beamed and glanced at his watch. "That's it, Joe—great idea. I don't have a case 'til one o'clock. I can talk to Dr. Hollander this morning." He drained his coffee cup and grinned at Joe. "I agree, we can trust Hollander—he'll help us. The only problem is how in the world to convince him it's more than some hare-brained notion."

Joe left to join his team in the operating room and Jeremy headed for the Education office. Hollander's reception room was small and wood-paneled, decorated in conservative style with splashes of deep red and dark green here and there. Bookshelves were everywhere, with photos and mementoes scattered among the books. Hollander's secretary was working at a keyboard on the console behind her desk, her back toward the entry. A pair of transcribing headphones creased her flaxen hair.

Jeremy knocked on the woman's desk. "Good morning, Miss Shannon."

Startled, she jumped away from the keyboard and whirled around. "Dr. Becker. I didn't hear you come in."

"I know you didn't. Sorry about that. I didn't mean to sneak up on you."

Colleen Shannon removed the headphones and arranged her hair. She flashed a coy smile in Jeremy's direction. "You can sneak up on me anytime you want to."

Jeremy laughed. "How've you been, Colleen? I don't think I've seen you since the surgery department's Christmas party."

"That was a great party. I just loved seeing all of you surgeons relax for a change. You're all so-o-o much fun when you let your hair down."

"I'm glad you had a good time." He smiled, recalling how tipsy she'd gotten. "Listen, Colleen, I need to see Dr. Hollander. Is he in?"

"He's in, but he's really busy with a report for the trustees." She waved toward the transcribing machine behind her. "That's what I was working on—the first part of it." She glanced toward her boss's door. "He's got to finish it this morning."

"I need to tell him about something really important. Can't you get me in for a few minutes?"

Colleen batted her large green eyes. "I'd love to help you, Jeremy, but Dr. Hollander would kill me. He told me not to interrupt him for anything."

Jeremy decided two could play at the game of flirtation. He leaned close and lowered his voice to a stage whisper. "Colleen, I'll make sure you get a special invitation to this year's Christmas party. I know a guy who'd be real happy to see you there."

Her pretty face twisted into a frown. "I don't know...."

"Just ask him. Tell him it's very important—important to the whole hospital. If he says no, I'll leave you alone."

"Well...okay, Jeremy, I'll ask him." Shaking her head, she got up slowly and started toward Hollander's office. "But no promises…."

Colleen disappeared inside, returning a few minutes later. She winked and left the office door open. She mouthed the words, "Christmas party," then motioned Jeremy toward the open door with a toss of her head.

He heard Charles Hollander's voice from inside the office. "Come on in, Becker. This better be important, or you and my secretary are both in big trouble."

When Jeremy walked in Hollander waved him to a chair near the desk. "I have to present the quarterly Education Report to the Board of Trustees at eleven. This is the first chance I've had to put the finishing touches on it."

"The Board meets today?" A poorly defined idea began to move around inside Jeremy's head. Bulls eye, he thought. Hard to beat that as a direct line to hospital authorities.

"Yes. At eleven." He glanced at his wrist watch and tapped a stack of papers on the desk. "So what's important enough that you had to interrupt me? Get on with it."

"I apologize for interrupting, but this really is important." He squinted at Hollander, then said, "It's about the unexpected deaths we've been having."

Hollander removed his half-frame glasses and laid them on the desk. "Okay, Becker. You've got my attention. Now tell me the rest of it."

"Well, I believe several patients have died under unusual circumstances in the past few weeks. Events leading to their deaths were strangely similar. I believe it's more than a coincidence."

"What on earth are you talking about, Becker?"

"I told my father about all of this when he was here recently. He convinced me something unusual is going on—something dangerous. I think you know he asked Joe Monteleone to review the patients' charts. Thanks for your help with that, by the way."

"No problem. I can't imagine Mr. Lockhart not allowing a member of the house staff to review the chart of any of our patients." He looked at Jeremy and asked, "Did Joe come up with anything?"

"Yes sir, we think he did." Jeremy hesitated while Hollander put on his glasses. "Each of the patients had volunteered for clinical safety trials of one of the experimental HIV protocols and—"

"That's not unusual, Becker. What else did Joe find?" Eyebrows raised, Hollander peered over his glasses. "Had the patients actually started any experimental treatment? We might want to discontinue those particular protocols until we learn more."

"No, sir. They were all enrolled and they all had the preliminary lab work, but none of them had started treatment. It's the clinical events leading to their deaths that we're worried about—they were all so similar."

Hollander looked at his watch. "We're not getting anywhere, Becker. Tell me what was similar about the deaths, but make it quick."

Good, Jeremy mused. Got him interested—he's involved. "All of the patients had practically recovered from whatever brought them in the hospital in the first place. Every one of 'em became ill very suddenly with a clinical picture like septic shock. Then, Dr. Hollander, each patient died within a couple of hours." He paused, let his words sink in. "The autopsies found no specific cause of death for any of them."

Hollander ran his hand through his thick white hair. "I agree that all sounds odd, Becker. But why is it so urgent? You said the patients died over a period of several weeks."

Now, Jeremy thought. Push it to the hilt. He stood up and leaned over Hollander's desk. "There is one new development. I believe there's a conspiracy involving members of the hospital staff that has something to do with the deaths of those patients."

Silence filled the room.

Hollander slid his glasses down on his nose and looked over them at Jeremy. He spoke softly. "Do you realize what you're suggesting? That's a very serious accusation."

"I know it's serious. That's why I'm here. I have reason to believe there's an surprising relationship between a hospital worker and someone in the research lab, a relationship that may be linked to the deaths of our patients."

Jeremy sat down again and summarized his suspicions about Guidry and Hebert. He told Hollander about stumbling upon their late night meeting. "They were arguing," he said, "practically fighting in a dark corner of a bar in the Quarter." He decided not to volunteer exactly which bar it was.

Hollander took off his glasses again and put them on top of his unfinished report. He looked directly at Jeremy. "Listen, it's almost ten now. I'm due at the Board meeting in less than an hour, but I don't like what you've told me so far. I want to hear the rest of it, but it'll have to be later."

"Good. You name the time." Jeremy stood up and glanced at his watch. "I should be finished in the operating room about five. You could page me whenever you're free after that."

"All right. I'll do that." Hollander walked around his desk, took Jeremy by the elbow and guided him toward the office door. "You may be onto something serious here. Don't discuss it with anyone else until we talk again. You were right to bring it to me."

Hollander stopped at the door and scratched his head. "Maybe I'll mention it to the Trustees.... No, that's not a good idea, not yet. No use to get everybody excited." He laughed. "The lawyers would go crazy with this wouldn't they?"

"Really." Jeremy smiled and turned to leave. "Thanks, Dr. Hollander. Sorry I had to interrupt you."

"Perhaps your father's right," Hollander said in low voice, almost like he was speaking to himself. "There could be danger." He turned to Jeremy. "I'll page you after five o'clock."

❖❖❖

36

President's Orders

When Jeremy left Dr. Hollander's office in the quiet administration wing of the hospital he saw his number flashing on the overhead panel of the silent paging system. He stopped in the lobby and answered from a staff telephone at the information desk. He'd missed a call from his father's office in Beaumont. Preferring privacy to return the call, he took an elevator to his fourteenth floor sleeping room.

"Hello, Dad. I just got your message."

"Good morning, Jere. How're you feeling? Getting back into your work routine?"

"I'm fine. No problems at all." He hesitated. "Listen, I'm glad you called. Joe and I've uncovered a new twist in the business about the hospital deaths."

"I have some news, too. But tell me what you've discovered first."

He told his father about the death of the virologist in the ER. "He had a bad auto crash, but none of his injuries should've been fatal. He responded more like septic shock—same as the other patients who've died. Didn't make a bit of sense to me."

"Fits right in with what I've learned," Dr. Becker said. "The whole thing may be more dangerous than I thought."

"What are you talking about?"

"In a minute. What else have you and Joe discovered?"

Uh oh, Jeremy thought. Here it comes. His father had urged him not to discuss any of these events with the hospital leaders, and now he had to tell him about talking to Hollander. He moved the receiver to his other ear. "We may have stumbled onto a connection between a housekeeping worker at the hospital and the HIV research lab. Looks like it could be related to the deaths, but it's definitely a hospital issue. Joe and I felt we had to take it to the senior staff here at Charity."

No sound came over the line. Nothing but total silence.

"I knew you'd say something like that," Jeremy said.

"I asked you not to involve anybody over there. Who did you talk to? Not that fool Lockhart, I hope."

"No, Dad, I wouldn't do that—I know how you feel about him. I went over the whole thing this morning with the Education Director."

"Who's in Education now? I hope it's somebody we can trust?"

"I think it is. It's Dr. Hollander—Charles Hollander. Do you know him?"

"Yes, I do. I've known Charles for a long time. He's a good man. If you had to talk to anybody over there, I'm glad you picked him. What's he going to do?"

"Nothing, yet. We're supposed to get together again late this afternoon. I'm pretty sure he'll want to start some kind of investigation."

"Ask him to keep it low key, Jeremy. The whole thing may be bigger than we expected—we ought to keep all the investigating in one place." He paused. "And that brings me to my news. Senator Randall called me this morning. He needs to get firsthand information about what's going on at Charity. He wants to talk to you in person. He's getting here tomorrow and we need you to come to Beaumont."

"You know I can't get away, Dad. Couldn't I just talk to him by phone?"

"I don't believe that'll work, son, he wants a sworn deposition. He asked me to arrange a meeting for the three of us, and he'd like it to be in Beaumont—or at least somewhere in Texas. He's particular about staying in his own jurisdiction."

Jeremy picked up a desk calendar and shook his head. "There's no way I can do that. Not after just being away for two weeks."

Dr. Becker laughed. "I told Warren you'd say that, but I promised I'd try. He said the three of us should meet on the sly in New Orleans if you can't get away—wants us to set it up for tomorrow night."

"How can we do that? There're no evening flights from Beaumont to New Orleans."

"Senator Randall's got access to a plane. A charter."

"Really? He must have found something pretty important. What's going on?"

"I'm not sure yet. Warren asked that you make a reservation at a place called the Cypress Club. It's one of those executive waiting areas at the airport. We need privacy, and Warren wants to be incognito, so reserve a private conference room in your name. There could be five or six of us altogether. It's a private club, so the HIV restrictions won't be a problem."

"How can I make the reservation? I'm not a member of the Cypress Club."

"Warren thought of that, but he doesn't want the reservation in his name for the public record. He gave me a code number—write this down."

"Okay, I'm ready."

"Speak to the club manager, a Mr. Singh, and give him code number 62-5450. Make sure the reservation's in your name, with all the charges to go on your credit card. I'll pay you for it later."

"Okay. What about a hotel? Will you be staying more than one night?"

"We won't be staying at all. We'll just meet with you then fly back to Beaumont. Reserve the conference room for the whole evening. We'll meet you there at nine o'clock."

Jeremy shook his head and chuckled. "I'm pretty impressed with Senator Randall's cloak and dagger stuff. Sounds like you're turning into a regular detective yourself."

After a long pause Dr. Becker said, "It's not a joke, Jeremy. You need to treat this information and the plans for our meeting with absolute confidence. No one must know. Not even Charles Hollander."

"All right. I won't discuss it." But a new thought popped into his head. "Listen, I think I should bring Barbara to the meeting. She knows more about the patients who died on the medicine wards than I do. She's involved in the whole thing anyway."

Jeremy sensed reluctance. Finally, his father said, "Okay. No harm in that, I guess. It might be good for Warren to hear two sides of the hospital story. Yes, do ask Barbara. Maybe Joe Monteleone could come, too."

"Joe's on duty tomorrow, Dad, but I'm pretty sure Barbara can come with me." He waited. "You were going to tell me what Senator Randall discovered."

"Oh, yes. Warren told me he's found pretty solid evidence of a long-standing financial link between one of your lab's Regional Directors and a congressman from Thibodaux."

"Thibodaux? Are you talking about Marshall Boudreaux? Remember, we heard about him at the lab briefing."

"Yes. Marshall Boudreaux and Congressman Pierre Legrande."

Jeremy stood up and walked to the end of the telephone cord. "I've heard of Representative Legrande. He must have been in Congress for twenty years."

"Longer than that, I think."

"Why does it surprise you if he has business connections with Boudreaux? They're from the same town. It doesn't sound unusual to me."

"There's more to it than a business connection. Warren didn't say much more than that—I'd rather he tell you the rest of it tomorrow night."

Jeremy shrugged. "Okay. If you say so. I'll set up everything on this end. Shall I call you to confirm it?"

"No need for that. Just let me know if you have a problem—otherwise we'll meet you at the airport at nine o'clock."

Jeremy hung up the phone and sat for several minutes, trying to fully understand the things he'd just heard from his father. All of a sudden he realized he might have put Dr. Hollander in a very awkward position. Shit, Marshall Boudreaux was on the hospital's Board of Trustees. He'd be at that meeting. If Hollander brought up the things Jeremy had told him...Jesus....

He jerked up the phone and dialed Hollander's office number. Busy. He looked at his watch. Ten fifty-eight. He dialed again. Still busy.

Gotta stop him. Damn phone! Goddamn busy signal! Maybe he could get down there in time. The frigging elevators would be too slow.

He raced into the hall, down the stairs to the first floor and on to the Education office. It was three past eleven. The secretary was on the telephone. "...early lunch. My boss is at the Trustees meeting, and I thought—"

Breathless, Jeremy tried to get her off the phone. "Colleen—we've got to stop—Dr. Hollander. Has he left—for the meeting?"

She put the phone on her desk. "He left fifteen minutes ago, Jeremy. What's the matter? Why are you breathing like that?"

"I ran down here—from the fourteenth floor." He tried to slow his breathing. "I've got to talk to Dr. Hollander. Call him at the meeting."

"I can't. There's no way to reach him there. What's wrong anyway?"

"I can't tell you that, Colleen. Trust me, I've got to talk to him before the Trustees meeting starts."

"That's impossible, Jeremy. The Chairman of the Board made them take the phones out of the meeting room. He won't even let 'em bring their pagers—said he was tired of interruptions and wasted time." She glanced at the clock on her desk. "The meeting's already started. There's no way to reach Dr. Hollander until it's over."

"There's got to be a way. I'm going over there." He headed for the door, then turned back and said, "Give me an envelope, quick."

Looking puzzled, Colleen handed him an envelope from her desk drawer.

Jeremy tore down the halls to the opposite end of Charity's main building, then sped along the covered walkway leading to an older red-brick buildings flanking Claiborne Avenue. He ran into the foyer of the old John Dibert TB building, but he was stopped by a security guard at the entrance to the executive conference room.

"I'm Dr. Becker. I need to go in please."

"Do you have a pass for the meeting?"

"No, I'm not going to the meeting. I have an urgent message for Dr. Hollander."

The guard checked the roster on his clipboard. "Dr. Charles Hollander?"

"Yes. I need to speak to him right away."

"I can't let you do that. Orders from the Board president."

Jeremy protested. "There's gotta be some way to get a message to him."

"I can give him a written message."

"Great. Just a minute." Jeremy pulled a three-by-five card out of his pocket and wrote:

> Dr. Hollander:
> URGENT that you not discuss suspicions with Board of Trustees. Will explain later.
> J. Becker

He sealed the card in Colleen's envelope, wrote Hollander's name on it and handed it to the guard. The man saluted with the envelope, but he made no move to enter the conference room.

"Aren't you gonna take it in?" Jeremy asked. "I'm waiting for his answer."

"Can't. Not right now. I have to wait 'til they take a break."

"What...?"

The guard shrugged. "Sorry, Board President's orders."

❖❖❖

37

OUTMANEUVERED

HOLLANDER FELT PRETTY GOOD ABOUT HIS QUARTERLY REPORT by the time he headed to the trustees' meeting. Still fifteen minutes to go and he was familiar enough with his data to present it credibly, though he had given up on his usual printed handout. Colleen had made some graphics for the overhead projector, and he felt comfortable about fielding the trustees' questions—they'd just have to get along without a printed copy of his report this time.

These Board meetings were a chore anyway, a political necessity Hollander did not enjoy. Switching from surgical practice to education had meant a sizable reduction in his income, but he was now an educator, and what he liked best was teaching a few medical students the art of surgery at a patient's bedside or in a small conference room with an x-ray view box.

Walking to the meeting Hollander found it hard to keep his mind on the report. He couldn't get away from the worrisome things Jeremy Becker had told him. Unexpected deaths, conspiracy—dangerous ideas. Then, in the Board Room's foyer, he was jolted him back to reality when the security guard grabbed him by the arm before he entered the meeting room.

"Need to see your pass, Doctor."

"Pass? Oh yes." He showed the man a laminated photo ID coded for access to certain executive functions, including the trustees' meetings. Inconvenient precautions—damned inconvenient. Necessary though, he guessed, after that bomb scare last year. The entire Board of Trustees had threatened to resign unless security was beefed up for their meetings. Our society demands too much, Hollander fretted. Far too much protection from one another. Whatever happened to trust?

He joined twenty or so men and women standing around the anteroom in groups of two or three, all of them busy with small talk and coffee while waiting for the chairman to begin the meeting. He saw several others in white coats—like himself, senior members of the medical staff. The trustees all wore conservative business suits, all but the archbishop in his clerical garb.

Hollander respected the trustees—they were totally supportive of the medical center. All of them were influential people, community leaders, movers and shakers who guided the directions of business and commerce and religion in New Orleans.

A well-dressed woman with gray hair sat at a small oval table in the center of the anteroom, pouring from a silver coffee service. Hollander didn't recognize her, probably somebody from the wives' auxiliary. He returned her smile and took the cup of coffee she offered.

He was reluctant to say very much in this place about the things Jeremy had told him, but he felt obliged to share the problem with somebody. Admittedly, the whole thing was pure speculation, but he could share it carefully—get other ideas about the best way to handle it. He spotted a political reporter from *The Times-Picayune* on the opposite side of the room—with that guy here any discussion would have to be circumspect. There'd be hell to pay if he got wind of Jeremy's story.

Hollander thought about just turning the whole thing over to Security, getting the police involved. No…there may be nothing to it. He needed to hear the rest of the story. Lockhart would be at this meeting...maybe he'd talk to him. The administrator was not somebody he'd normally ask for advice, but maybe he should mention it to him, see how he reacted.

He had no trouble spotting Lockhart. As usual, the administrator's clothes were the most conspicuous in the room. Shoulders padded, lapels a little wider than most, necktie coordinating the rainbow of colors he always wore. Hollander shook his head. That guy must have a closet full of those blazers—every one of 'em a different color. Today it was burgundy, not a subdued hue, but bright, more like cranberry. With it he wore gray trousers, a gray and burgundy paisley tie with a few yellow lightning bolts running through it—and a bright yellow shirt.

Balancing his coffee cup, Hollander threaded his way through the crowd to reach Lockhart at one end of the room. Looked like he was talking to one of the trustees. Ah good, it was Marshall Boudreaux—he'd be the right man to hear about the residents' concerns.

Boudreaux was a tall man, well over six feet. He tended toward the stocky side, but that was disguised by the expert tailoring of his double-breasted, navy blue pinstripe suit. Hollander knew Boudreaux considered Charity Hospital his own private turf—he liked to hear all the dirt. Too bad he wasn't alone. Boudreaux was somebody he wouldn't mind confiding in.

Pleased with his luck at making it through the crowd with his coffee still in the cup, Hollander reached the two men just as Lockhart threw both of his arms outward in some exuberant gesture. But for Hollander's deft movement, the blazer would have been cranberry with a coffee sleeve. "Careful there, Larry. Almost got you."

Lockhart acknowledged his arrival with an imperial nod. Hollander turned to the older man. "Morning, Mr. Boudreaux."

Boudreaux smiled and spoke with the practiced voice of a senior executive. "Good morning to you, Dr. Hollander. Always nice to see you at our meetings. Have your report today, do you?"

"Yes sir, the usual quarterly summary, but there's something else—a potential problem I need to make Larry aware of. Sorry if I interrupted your conversation."

"No interruption," Boudreaux said. "None at all. Do you mind if I listen in, or is it a private matter?"

Lockhart peered down his long nose. "Charles, there's really no reason to bother Mr. Boudreaux with hospital trivia. I'm sure we can solve your problem—call me this afternoon."

Hollander read Lockhart's body language: Get lost! I'm trying to make points with an important man. I don't need somebody like you to fuck it up.

Boudreaux put his hand on Lockhart's arm. "It's okay, Larry. I like to know what's going on in the trenches." He turned to Hollander and smiled again. "What's this problem you wanted to talk about?"

"Well, let's just call it a potential problem. I'm not sure how serious it actually is, but one of the house staff told me about—"

"Charles, this is not the time for a problem with the house staff," Lockhart said.

Hollander glanced at the pompous administrator with a look that would freeze sea water, then he smiled at Boudreaux. "It's not actually a problem with the house staff. One of the residents thinks we're having a run of unexpected deaths."

Lockhart raised his eyebrows and drew in a breath, but this time he kept quiet.

"Do you think there's anything to it?" Boudreaux asked.

"I haven't decided yet, but I don't think I can just dismiss it. He's a level-headed young man, a senior resident with mature judgment. He's never been a trouble maker. Some of the things he told me did sound a little suspicious."

"Suspicious of what, Hollander? Don't beat around the bush." Boudreaux glanced toward the reporter, then put his arm around Hollander's shoulders and guided him to an empty corner of the room. Lockhart stuck to them like a barnacle on a river piling, and the three moved together through the crowd.

Boudreaux detoured by the serving table to return his coffee cup, then said, "Now tell us what you're talking about. It sounds like something I need to hear."

Hollander told them some of the things he'd heard from Jeremy, describing the series of deaths among the hospital's patients and the medical circumstances surrounding them.

Boudreaux held up his hand. "Hold on there, I don't understand all that medical talk. Are you convinced the patients didn't die of whatever brought 'em to the hospital in the first place?"

Lockhart joined in. "I agree. They must have died of their underlying illnesses. Don't you think that's more likely, Charles?"

"No. I don't think that at all. I believe a group of patients with different illnesses all died of some unknown cause that gave each of one them a surprisingly similar clinical picture at the time of death."

"Could it have been AIDS?" Boudreaux asked. "Obviously, all of them were HIV-positive."

"If they died of AIDS, Mr. Boudreaux, it's an entirely new pattern of the disease— something that hasn't yet been described in the medical literature."

Boudreaux pressed his lips together and nodded his head.

Lockhart looked sideways at Hollander, watching Boudreaux closely while he spoke. "Does this have anything to do with those medical records you insisted had to be reviewed?"

"Yes, it does. Those patients were the first ones. Those deaths triggered the suspicions in the first place."

"So, that's it. It's part of that ruckus Dr. Becker wanted to stir up. I should have known he'd—"

"Dr. Becker?" Boudreaux said. "Who's Becker?"

Lockhart shot Boudreaux a smug grin. "Dr. Becker is a practitioner from Beaumont. It was his son who was injured in that quarrel with a patient's family."

"Yes, I remember the incident. How's the boy doing?" They both looked at Hollander.

"He seems to have recovered fully. He's back at work. He's the one who brought this to my attention, in fact." Hollander hesitated and lowered his voice. "There's more. I haven't told you all of it. Jeremy Becker is convinced there's a conspiracy in the hospital that's related in some way to all of the deaths."

Boudreaux looked at the floor. He straightened his tie and shifted his weight.

Lockhart said, "Surely you agree this whole thing is ridiculous, Charles." He flashed Boudreaux a reassuring look. "Our residents can be very imaginative. This must be some fantasy from their exhausted minds. Everybody knows how hard they work on the surgical service, so it's easy—"

Boudreaux looked up. "Surgical service you say? Who else is involved in this, Dr. Hollander? Who else knows about it?"

"I don't think the whole service is involved," Hollander said. "As far as I know, Jeremy Becker and one other surgery resident are the only ones who suspect anything out of the ordinary. Becker told me about it this morning."

Marshall Boudreaux gazed across the crowded room, then turned to Hollander and said, "Who's the other resident?"

"His name is Monteleone. Joseph Monteleone. Why?"

Boudreaux took a leather-bound note pad and a gold pen from his breast pocket. He wrote the two residents' names and returned the pad to his jacket.

Agitated, Lockhart pulled at the collar of his shirt.

"Please understand me," Hollander said, "this may be nothing at all. On the other hand, it could become a big problem for the whole medical center. That's why I wanted you to know about it, Larry. I plan to start looking into it this afternoon."

Boudreaux's face twisted. He scratched his jaw with manicured fingernails. "Maybe you don't want to do that, Dr. Hollander. The two of you can't even agree whether there is a problem. There's nothing to gain by an official investigation. Not yet. It could even be embarrassing, like...well, like crying wolf. There's no point to it."

Lockhart bounced from one foot to the other. Hollander waited. Boudreaux was an experienced corporate manager, and he wanted to hear what the man had to say.

Boudreaux touched Hollander's shoulder. "Why don't we just let this be a private conversation? I can check a few things myself, unofficially. Anything more formal could become a matter of public record, you know—let me take care of this one. If there's anything to it, we can get an official investigation going when we're on firmer ground. If not, we can just forget the whole thing." He chuckled and nodded toward the reporter. "That way, if it's a false alarm, we can avoid embarrassing the hospital."

Lockhart nodded his agreement.

Hollander was doubtful. "I think I should at least look into the medical aspects of it."

He knew Boudreaux was a man long accustomed to directing others. He stood quietly while Boudreaux smiled broadly and said, "Let me do it for you. You're busy enough running the residency programs. I'll get my people to check out the whole thing, then we can talk again."

The men and women around them began to move into the conference room, and Boudreaux turned to join the other trustees. "Let's go in. I'll get back to you on this in a day or two."

Puzzled, Hollander walked into the conference room. Lockhart took his elbow and leaned close. "Charles, why on earth did you bring up all that bullshit with a man like Boudreaux? Surely you don't believe there's anything to it."

"I'm not sure about that, Larry. Not at all sure."

The meeting began with the usual drone of parliamentary procedures and routine reports. Hollander's attention wandered. The chairman reached the end of a long report of bed occupancy rates and hospital mortality for each month of the preceding quarter. "Looks like the medical staff is doing its usual excellent job," he said. "The census remains high, the length of stay is not excessive and the overall mortality rate appears stable." He looked around the table. "You each have a copy of this report. Any questions? Comments?"

Boudreaux raised his hand. "I have a question."

He waited for the chairman's nod, then said, "I'm interested in these death rates. I agree the figures look good, but this report shows only the past three months. How does it stack up against the previous quarter? Seems to me the mortality rates have been about the same for a long time. Do you have any of the older figures there?"

The chairman did have that information, and the recorder duly noted the board's agreement that there appeared to be no recent increase in the hospital's death rate. Hollander saw Boudreaux glance at him. He could not interpret the man's expression, though he was certain he saw the slightest lift of his eyebrows.

Finally, it was time for Hollander's education report. His presentation took less than ten minutes, then he answered questions for another five. Afterward, he tried to position himself to leave the room quickly, but he failed—the trustees slowed him down. Chairs pushed back, chatting with one another, the crowd made it difficult to move toward the door. Delayed anyway, Hollander decided to find Boudreaux and make a definite appointment to meet again. They had unfinished business.

Boudreaux was not in his chair, not visible in the crowd. Where was he? There, huddled in the corner with Lockhart—looked like an animated discussion they were having. Boudreaux was doing the talking, Lockhart listening most of the time. Lockhart's movements looked like his usual overreaction when he was under attack. What the hell...what was going on with those two?

Whatever, this was not the best time to discuss anything with Boudreaux. Hollander felt he needed to do more than just wait for the man to call him, but that was all he could do now. He was outmaneuvered by the man he'd picked as a sounding board. He'd burned all his bridges.

Frustrated, Hollander left the meeting room, but the security guard stopped him again. "What now?" he asked. "I don't need a pass to get out of here do I?"

"No, Dr. Hollander. You don't need a pass, but I have a message for you. One of the residents left it right after the meeting started. He said it was urgent, but y'all never did take a break, so this is the first chance I had to give it to you."

After reading Jeremy's brief note Hollander rushed back to his office. He waved the note at his secretary and said, "Colleen, call Jeremy Becker and set up a time for me to meet with him this afternoon. The sooner the better."

❖❖❖

38

THE CYPRESS CLUB

THE NEXT DAY'S WORKLOAD WAS BUSIER THAN JEREMY expected. It was after seven when he and the team finished evening rounds. In less than two hours his father and Senator Randall would be at the airport. If he hurried he and Barbara could still get there before them, but it'd be mighty close.

He bolted off the elevator on the fourteenth floor and ran down the hall. Thinking Joe was in the room, he tried the door at running speed, but the door was locked and he crashed into it. Fumbling in the pockets of his hospital coat, he remembered his key ring was pinned to the scrubs he was still wearing. He pulled off the coat and felt along the waist of his loose-fitting scrub pants. Where...? There. He turned the room key in the lock and raced inside.

Throwing clothes wherever they fell, he hit the shower without slowing down. Shit, he'd left his notes at the apartment, notes showing the chronology of patient deaths. His deposition wouldn't be complete without those notes—he'd have to stop by there on the way to Barbara's.

Fifteen minutes later he had showered and shaved, and he walked out of the bathroom toweling his wet hair. Better call Barb, he decided. Let her know he was running late.

"Want me to fix you a sandwich to eat in the car?" she asked.

"Thanks—that's nice, but don't bother."

"Okay. I've got to make it an early night this time. I have a charge nurses' meeting at the crack of dawn."

"Yeah, I have an early case, too. I'll try to see you by eight-fifteen. Could you meet me out front?"

Jeremy dressed in khakis and an open shirt and threw a cotton sweater over his shoulders, then reached in the drawer for his billfold and.... Whoa, where in the hell were those keys? Oh yeah, probably left 'em in the lock.

He gave his hair a final brush then headed for the door, ready to leave, but his keys were not in the lock after all. Baffled now, he returned to the room and searched the dresser again. He picked up his discarded clothes and checked every pocket. He looked on the desk, on the bedside table, all around the floor, even in the bathroom. No keys.

Now what? Without the damn keys he couldn't do anything. No car keys, no apartment keys. Hell, he couldn't even lock the door to the sleeping room.

Joe....he was on duty that night, maybe still making rounds. He could page Joe, use his keys, borrow his car. No, paging took too long—quicker to go down to his ward.

Lucky at last, Jeremy found Joe and his team exactly where he thought they'd be, in their examining room going over their patients' x-rays. "Hi, guys. Sorry to interrupt your rounds, Joe, but I need your help."

"No problem," Joe said. "What's the matter?"

"You know my plans for tonight?" He hesitated until Joe nodded. "I'm late and I really need to get going, but I've lost my car keys. They're in the room somewhere, but I can't find the damn things."

"Don't you keep an extra set at the apartment?"

"My apartment keys are on the same ring."

Joe chuckled. "Sounds like you're in big trouble. Listen, we're about finished here, one of us can take you...." He shook his head. "No, no. Better idea. Why don't you just use my car tonight? I sure won't need it—we've already got a couple of emergencies on the books. Use my keys for the apartment, too. We can find yours in the morning."

"That'd be great, Joe. Do you mind?"

"Not at all." Joe opened his coat and touched a single key pinned to his scrub shirt. "This room key's the only one I've got with me—the others are in the closet. Look on the hanger with the clothes I wore to work this morning. This room key won't help you."

Returning to Room 1408, Jeremy was annoyed to discover he'd left the door wide open. He found Joe's keys in the closet, exactly where he said they'd be. Without thinking, he checked the dresser top one last time on the way out. Wait a minute—his missing keys were there. Right there on the dresser. Come on, he'd been in a hurry, but this was more like dementia or something. Oh well, things could only get better now. He left Joe's keys on the dresser and rushed back to the elevator.

It was nearly eight by the time he pulled out of the hospital garage. Downtown traffic had thinned for the day, and he made it to the Quarter in record time. He hurried through the courtyard and unlocked the apartment. As he rushed inside the dark room, the white shag rug near the door caught his eye. Good, Joe got it back from the cleaners. Great roommate. He grabbed his notes from the desk, spun around and headed back through the courtyard without slowing down.

Back in the Miata, he drove out Esplanade toward City Park. Eight-twenty—they'd never make it. Barbara's apartment was in a modern complex on Bayou Saint John. He spotted her waiting out front as he pulled up to the curb. Barbara let herself in the passenger seat and gave him a quick kiss.

Jeremy turned off the engine and unfastened his seat belt. He leaned across the console and took Barbara in his arms and grinned. "Listen, I've been running for the past two hours. Time to slow down for the important stuff." He kissed her then, his tongue exploring her lips.

"Hmmm, hello," Barbara said. "Can I get in the car again and try that one more time?"

"I'd love to try it all night long, but I think we better get going. Dad and the senator will be there at nine."

The expressway to Moissant Airport was congested, and it was five past nine when they reached the terminal. "Any idea where the Cypress Club is?" Jeremy asked.

"No, I thought you knew."

He took Barbara's hand and pulled her toward the nearest ticket counter. "Let's ask somebody."

With directions, they finally found the club in an out-of-the-way corner of the terminal, just outside the security gate of a boarding concourse. As many times as Jeremy had used that concourse, he'd never noticed the Cypress Club. "Doesn't look like much, does it?"

The ordinary looking wooden door had no markings except for a small sign showing the club's name and Private—Members and Guests Only. Jeremy pushed the door open and led Barbara into a foyer which required a quick left turn into a very different kind of space, a large, relaxing space which suggested there'd be no more hurrying tonight.

A sweeping expanse of silver-gray carpet pulled their eyes across a warmly-lighted room to a glass wall that overlooked a taxiway with planes moving about like silent ghosts. The lounge smelled clean and fresh. It was as quiet as a library except for soft tones of chamber music that drifted from hidden speakers.

Groupings of leather upholstered sofas and lounge chairs were separated from a few reading tables by large green plants in burnt orange ceramic pots. Several people, none of them together apparently, sat here and there reading, some nursing coffee cups or cocktail glasses on nearby end tables.

A svelte youngish woman wearing a gray and burnt orange uniform approached them. "Good evening. Welcome to the Cypress Club. May I have your membership card so I can sign you in."

"My name is Jeremy Becker. I was told to ask for Mr. Singh."

The woman smiled. "You're lucky. He's working late tonight." She asked them to wait, then returned a few minutes later with a tall, slender, dark-skinned man wearing a male version of the gray and burnt orange outfit.

"Hello, Dr. Becker. I am Roger Singh." Shaking Jeremy's hand, then Barbara's, Singh welcomed them like royal guests, bowing slightly as he spoke with a clipped British accent. "Your guests got here a short while ago. Come, I'll show you where they are."

He turned and led them toward the far corner of the lounge. "I ordered coffee and a tray of sandwiches for you. Would you like anything more?"

Jeremy winked at Barbara. "I don't think so. I'll ask the others."

Singh opened the door of a private conference room, then stood aside to wave them in. "Your telephone is there on the side table. Just touch eight if you need anything—bar service, steno support, anything like that. The loo is right through that door. We won't disturb you unless you call."

Jeremy's father, Senator Randall, and a younger man sat in chairs grouped on one side of a modern coffee table placed on a burnt orange area rug. A gray leather sofa opposite the chairs separated the sitting area from a conference table surrounded by six executive chairs. A bookcase wall and the restroom door Singh had pointed out were on the far side of the table. The main lounge's glass wall extended into this room as well, but here, sheer drapes covered the glass.

"Here they are," said the senator, as the three men got up and walked toward the door. Senator Randall was a handsome man in his early sixties. Taller than average, he still had a trim body, and his face was tanned. Wavy brown hair, thick and half-gray, barely touched the tops of his ears. It was neatly trimmed in a style that revealed not a single hair out of place. Though Jeremy hadn't seen the senator for several years, he remembered the lines about his eyes and mouth that could only have been shaped by a perpetual smile.

Jeremy introduced Barbara and learned the younger man was Chip

Daniels, an attorney who was a senior member of Senator Randall's staff.

"Did you have your second meeting with Charles Hollander?" Jeremy's father asked.

Jeremy nodded.

"Were you able to talk him out of starting an investigation?"

"I didn't have to," said Jeremy. "Marshall Boudreaux had already told him to let it alone."

The senator and Daniels exchanged a glance.

"How did Boudreaux get involved?" Dr. Becker asked. "What happened?"

Jeremy explained the unpredictable events that had triggered Hollander's discussion with Boudreaux, and told them of his own futile effort to warn Hollander before he reached the trustees' meeting. "I couldn't do anything about it. By the time I got your call, he was already at the meeting."

Jeremy's father loosened his tie and shook his head. "I'm sorry, Warren. Sounds like we've lost control of the situation."

Randall did not appear upset. "Don't worry about it. At least we know Boudreaux's aware somebody is suspicious. He'll think it's a low-level concern, something inside the medical center. Maybe we can get the evidence we need before he learns anybody else is involved."

The telephone rang, and everyone looked at Jeremy. "You'd better answer it," Senator Randall said. "The rest of us managed to get in here with only Roger Singh knowing who we were. I'd like to keep it that way."

It was Singh on the line. The sandwiches were ready. He brought them in with a large carafe of coffee and a tray of cups, then left the room. "What about Singh?" Jeremy asked. How do you know you can trust him?"

"We know Singh," Randall said. "He's done work for the Judiciary Committee in the past."

While the others poured coffee, Chip Daniels set up a tape recorder at one end of the conference table and laid several file folders beside it. He picked up his own cup then, and nodded to Randall. "All set, Senator."

Randall walked to the chair at the head of the table and took charge of the meeting with the ease of a man long accustomed to that role. "Jeremy, Barbara, I'd like you to sit here on either side of me so we can get the whole story on our tape. We may ask you some questions from time to time, but what we want is a clear understanding of the things you've been concerned about in the medical center. Just tell us about your patients."

"Okay to use my notes?" Jeremy asked.

"Sure. If you'll give us the notes afterward, we can make them part of the record." Randall looked at his watch. "Ready to get started? Don't rush your coffee, just bring the cups with you. This isn't a formal hearing. I do have to swear you in, but after that it'll just be a conversation among friends, okay?"

After taking the oath, Barbara and Jeremy retold every detail of the clinical events surrounding the patient deaths at Charity. Jeremy described the more recent cases, including the virologist who had died in the emergency room. He told about the routine of hospital patients volunteering for human toxicity trials for new HIV treatments, and the fact that the patients who'd died had all been volunteers.

Senator Randall took off his suit jacket, then refilled his cup and offered the carafe around the table. "Jeremy, are you suggesting the HIV drug trials are related to the deaths? What about that man who died in the emergency room? Was he a test subject?"

"He was not a test subject, but he did work at the HIV lab. His boss told me about a minor injury he'd sustained in a lab accident that same day, but there was nothing much to it. Just a small laceration on his hand—looked clean when I examined him. We cultured the wound at autopsy, but nothing's grown out. Not yet anyway."

"How long does a culture take?" Randall asked.

"The usual cultures, for bacteria, only take a couple of days, but a virus culture can take two months or more."

Daniels pulled a paper from one of the file folders. "You said he was a virologist, right?"

"Yes," Jeremy said. "Worked in the live virus section."

"Live virus...." Daniels scanned down the paper. "Is that Dr. Dan Hebert's area? Hebert's assistant chief of virology, isn't he?"

"That's right." Damn, Jeremy thought, these guys had really done their homework.

"Do you know Dr. Hebert?" Daniels asked.

"I met him a couple of weeks ago—when I toured the lab." Jeremy grinned at his father. "Dad can tell you about that. I also talked to Hebert when he came to the ER while we were working on that virologist from his section, then...." Should he mention what he saw at the bar?

"Then what?"

"Well, a few days later Joe and I—my roommate, Joe Monteleone and I ran across Dr. Hebert in a late-night meeting with a housekeeping worker from Charity. They didn't know we spotted 'em, but it looked odd to me—those two together. They were arguing about something."

Daniels took off his tortoise shell glasses and motioned toward the senator. "That's all I've got. You want to take it from here, Senator?"

Randall stood up and walked to the window and looked out into the night. "That's about it, then. What you've told us should tie down some of the loose ends." Turning back toward the conference table, he continued. "It is very important that no one learn about your involvement in our investigation. It could be dangerous for you if—"

The telephone rang again, reverberating on the hard table top and startling Jeremy. Eager to stop the noisy ringing, he hurried over to pick it up.

A strange, low-pitched voice spoke with an ominous inflection. "Is this Jeremy Becker?"

Jeremy wrinkled his brow and glanced at the others. "Who's calling please?"

"A friend of the senator. Are you Jeremy Becker?"

"Yes, I am. Who are you?"

"Sorry, Dr. Becker, I'm Senator Randall's pilot. He told me your meeting was hush-hush, so I wanted to be damn sure I had the right room before I mentioned his name. I need to speak to the senator if he's still there."

Jeremy waved the phone toward Randall. "It's your pilot calling for you." He tried to distance himself from the conversation, but he heard the senator chuckle and saw him look at his watch.

When Randall rejoined the group he put his hand on Jeremy's shoulder. "I was about to tell you I've been talking to the FBI. The Special-Agent-in-Charge for this district has put a team on stand-by for me. An agent by the name of Borgne...is that right, Chip?"

"Yes sir, Andy Borgne."

The senator nodded. "Borgne will contact you at the hospital when I give the go-ahead." He smiled at Barbara, gave Jeremy a pat on the shoulder, and motioned toward the restroom door. "Now, if you'll excuse me for a minute?" When he returned to the table, Randall stood next to Daniels and scanned the notes he'd made. "Did we miss anything, Chip?"

"No sir, the main thing we needed was the medical details." Daniels ran his finger along the notes. "I guess we should ask Jeremy where he saw Dr. Hebert meeting with that housekeeper—what was the housekeeper's name?"

"Guidry, Jeremy said. "Leonard Guidry. Joe and I saw those two at a bar in the Quarter."

Taking notes again, Daniels asked, "For the record, Jeremy, what was the name of the bar?"

"It was a place called The Eagle, on Governor Nicholls." When he spoke, Jeremy saw Barbara's eyes narrow for a brief instant.

❖❖❖

39

New Worries

Senator Randall stood up. "I believe that just about covers it for tonight." He nudged Daniels' arm. "Better pack up, Chip. That was our pilot on the phone. There's weather moving in. He wants to take off in half an hour." He waved the others toward the sitting area and put his hands on the shoulders of both Beckers. "I'm sorry you two didn't have much time for a visit, but I'm not one to gamble on marginal weather in small planes."

Jeremy filled everybody's coffee cup, then said, "Barbara and I are eager to hear what you've found, Senator Randall. Can't you tell us what's going on in Washington? What have you found that ties in with what we're seeing here? What was important enough to bring you all the way over here?"

Randall flashed a mischievous grin. "Well...I guess you know I've been asking a few questions. I'm looking for anything unusual about Charity Hospital, anything odd about your HIV Research Facility."

Finally, Barbara spoke up. "Senator, I haven't said very much tonight, but I think we need to know what's going on. Jeremy told me you might have discovered something important. Can't you tell us what it is?"

"I can tell you some of it. The rest is so speculative I'd rather not discuss it yet." He looked around the group. "I've discovered some interesting things about your man Marshall Boudreaux."

"He's pretty important around here," Jeremy said. "One of Charity's strongest advocates, from what I hear."

A gentle smile played at the corners of Randall's mouth. "Boudreaux may be more important that you know, Jeremy. He's a strong voice on your hospital's Board of Trustees, and I hear he likes to manipulate everyday management decisions. His pull in the state legislature keeps Charity's funds flowing from Baton Rouge, even when the budget is tight."

Jeremy picked up a sandwich and passed the tray to the others.

Senator Randall said, "Boudreaux's also chairman of the Board of Directors' Financial Committee at your research facility. Any idea what that means?"

Jeremy shook his head. "Well, no. Other than planning the budget—things like that."

"That's not all. He controls most of the money your lab spends. His committee oversees everything from travel and grants to supplies and equipment." He paused and looked around the group. "Discounting salaries and the appropriations to set up the regional labs, that's got to be over six hundred million dollars of federal funding every year. Boudreaux's managing every penny of it—and he does know how to manage it."

Jeremy coughed and put the sandwich down. "That's a lot of money, but surely you don't think Boudreaux's stealing from the lab. How could he do that? And why? He's already a rich man."

Randall squinted very slightly, almost imperceptibly. "Maybe not rich enough."

Jeremy raised his eyebrows. "Dad told me you discovered he's in some kind of partnership with a congressman."

Randall nodded. "That's right. Congressman Pierre Legrande."

"Help me understand why you're worried about that. They're from the same town—is their business unethical or something?"

"Theirs is not a normal business relationship, Jeremy. A lot of people on Capitol Hill have long suspected that Pierre Legrande has a hidden source of income, but nothing incriminating has ever surfaced."

"Boudreaux must be a pretty wealthy man," Barbara said. "Isn't it possible he's allowing the partnership to support the congressman as a senior partner?"

"Yes, that is possible," Randall said. "But I'm not sure Boudreaux could afford it. Congressman Legrande lives like a monarch. We don't know yet, but I believe we'll find Boudreaux could not afford it. I'm almost ready to subpoena his tax records, then I'll find out whether he has enough money to support Legrande's flamboyant life style."

"I don't understand what that has to do with our patients," Jeremy said. "We may be talking about murder, here. You don't think Boudreaux's involved in something like that, do you?"

"I can't help thinking it's all tied together. But my suspicions are circumstantial at best." Randall locked onto Jeremy's eyes. "I can't make a serious move until we've got a solid case—I can't afford to be wrong. That's where you two come in. Working with the FBI, inside the hospital, I'm betting you can turn up some hard evidence. I'm also betting Marshall Boudreaux and Pierre Legrande are involved in all of it. I need you to ferret out the missing pieces."

Jeremy drank the last of his coffee and put the cup on the table. "How can we do that? What do you want us to do?"

"I don't want you to do anything right now—not by yourselves. Wait to hear from the FBI. It won't be more than a day or two. And remember what I said about being careful. I'm sorry I have to be so mysterious about all this, but my warnings are serious. The danger is real."

After goodbyes, the three men departed for their flight to Beaumont. Alone with Barbara in the meeting room, Jeremy took another sandwich and offered her one. She shook her head, then looked at him for a long time without speaking.

"What's the matter?" he asked. "How do you feel about all this stuff?"

"Jeremy, isn't The Eagle a gay bar?"

"Yes. Why?"

"You didn't tell me you and Joe went to a gay bar."

"Wait a minute. I didn't intend to hide it from you—it just didn't seem important. Surely you don't think—"

"I don't know what to think, Jere. Don't forget what happened to me when I was married to Scott—I can't go through that again. Women don't know how to cope with that kind of competition, Jeremy. We know a few things to do when it's another woman, but if it's a man...."

"Sit down, Barbara. You're jumping the gun here. Going to that bar was completely innocent. Joe was celebrating, and he was overdue for a little fun. I let him talk me into going to The Eagle with him, but that's all there was to it."

"Do you mean that?"

"God's truth." He pulled her up into his embrace and nuzzled her ear. "Let's go to the apartment. I'll show you how true it is."

She melted into his arms, then laughed and rubbed her tears onto his neck. "Let's get out of this place. It's spooky after all that talk about danger and the FBI."

"I agree." Jeremy looked at his watch. "It's not too late, not even midnight yet. Come to Burgundy Street with me."

Barbara kissed him. "Not tonight, Jeremy. I need to go home."

"You're not going to worry about the bar thing are you?"

"No, forget it." She kissed him again.

Light rain began to fall before Jeremy's Miata reached the airport freeway. The first gusts of a northerly front blew an unseasonable chill across the flat terrain and, when they turned toward the city, Jeremy found Barbara's hand and pulled her as close as bucket seats would allow. As the car accelerated into the dark night Barbara reached for the dashboard and pushed the air control toward the setting for heat.

Rain was falling in earnest by the time they reached Barbra's apartment. It was coming down hard enough to remind Jeremy that much of the city was lower than Lake Ponchatrain and only the levee kept the Mississippi River out of the streets. He thought of the time-tested underground pumping system that pushed rainwater from the city into the lake and realized the pumps were made for nights like this one.

❖❖❖

40

A Deluge

SNUG IN THE PARKED CAR OUTSIDE HER APARTMENT, BARBARA AND Jeremy said a lingering goodnight. He tried again to convince her to go home with him, but she wouldn't budge on that. "We're both gonna get drenched anyway," he said. "Why don't we just do it together?"

Peering through the Miata's window, Barbara grinned and squeezed his thigh. "No, Jere, not tonight…maybe I can run fast between the drops to my front door."

Finally she gave him one last kiss and made a dash for it. Jeremy watched through the wet gusts until she was safely inside, then drove to the Quarter.

Street parking near his apartment, always difficult, seemed scarcer than usual in the downpour. He felt lucky to find a space on St. Ann, nearly two blocks away. It was still coming down hard—he knew he'd be soaked, so he decided to leave his shoes in the car. Shirt, too, along with his sweater and belt. They'd all be safe under the seat.

Without shoes and bare to the waist, he ran through the deluge. Waterlogged by the time he reached the corner of Burgundy, only one block short of the apartment, he hoped the pumps were all working. This storm had already dropped enough water to cause street flooding.

Then it happened. Too late to run out of the way, Jeremy saw both the muddy water filling the intersection and the car racing toward it—an old white Chrysler with rusty fenders and a sound system that pushed a loud bass beat into the narrow street. The Chrysler plowed into the huge puddle less than four feet from where Jeremy stood and red-brown muck instantly covered him from head to bare toe. "Bastard!" he yelled into the wet night, shooting a finger at the Chrysler's taillights.

He stopped then and stood in the rain, shaking his head. What were the odds? Must be a million to one against him and the only car in sight reaching that corner at exactly the same moment. No use to run now. He might as well enjoy it, let the rain wash off the mud.

Feeling like a ten-year-old, he splashed his feet through every puddle for the remaining block. In the brick-paved courtyard he hop-scotched across the mud that had washed from the planters and grinned, remembering a childhood rainy day when he had done something like that with his sister, Elaine. They'd caught hell for tracking mud in the house that day.

Finally inside the apartment, Jeremy closed the door and took off his wet trousers and briefs. He lighted the gas heater and opened the sofa bed, then slipped into a hot shower. Afterward, warm and dry, he abandoned the idea of making something hot to drink. Too much trouble, he decided. He'd forget about the kitchen, just go to bed.

Then, remembering the wet clothes he'd thrown on the floor, he walked to the door, but stopped short before he picked them up. Dammit—a muddy shoe print on the clean white rug. What a klutz. How had he managed that?

Jeremy touched the print. Still damp. Too late to worry about it anyway—better to brush it off in the morning after it dried. He tossed his wet clothes into the bathroom sink and dried the painted-brick floor with a towel, then crawled under the blanket.

Within minutes he was asleep. Moments later...no, longer, a squeaking, scraping sound forced its way into his subconscious. What was that? In a fleeting dream he saw the accordion door that closed off the kitchen. He dreamed a burly man holding out a police badge pulled the door open, and again he heard that scraping noise.

Suddenly, the reality of the sound he'd heard burst into Jeremy's consciousness and he woke up. Unnerved, he sat up in bed. Sounded like the rain had stopped. Patio gaslight flickered through the window. Except for his own breathing the room was silent.

Then, in the darkness, he spotted an unfamiliar shape, a shadow that looked like a large man crouched beside the desk. Jeremy sat motionless, barely breathing, watching. The shadow stood upright. The beat of Jeremy's own heart pounded in his ears. Damn, the shadow was a man, and he took a slow-motion step toward the bed.

"Who's there?" Jeremy shouted. "What do you want?"

No answer—silence filled the room. Flickering light from the window gave the scene a strobe-like appearance. The intruder crept closer to the bed, still in slow motion like a dream sequence. Then Jeremy spotted the knife in his hand, a large knife with a shiny blade that reflected the gaslight.

Jesus Christ, the guy was coming after him. Jeremy reached over his head, yanked a framed poster from the wall and hurled it toward the man as he raised his knife and lunged. A corner of the metal frame struck the intruder's shoulder. The knife ripped into the mattress beside Jeremy.

Jeremy rolled over and vaulted off the bed. He raced across the room and jerked the closet door open. The closet was dark—he couldn't see a damn thing. Without light, he'd never find the weapon he was looking for. Where in the hell was it? Where did he leave it? He stretched up to the top shelf and groped around. There—there it was. Hard polished wood. Solid, reassuring wood. His baseball bat.

The intruder seemed slow about pulling his knife blade from the mattress. He worked hard at it like it was stuck in the bed frame. By the time he freed it, Jeremy stood outside the closet whipping the bat through the air like a saber.

"Okay, you son of a bitch. What do you want? Come after me now." He heard the prowler's heavy breathing, saw his shoulders heave, smelled his own sour, fear-driven stink.

The man stepped into the flickering light near the window and Jeremy made out a beard, a dark, shaggy beard that covered most of his face—not a face he'd ever seen before. The intruder acted confused, glancing quickly around the room, squinting like he couldn't quite see where to go next, yet still homing in on Jeremy and the baseball bat.

Reassured by his attacker's hesitation, Jeremy edged sideways toward the kitchen. Keeping a wall near his back, he lashed the bat back and forth like an angry cat's tail. Gripping the hard shaft of wood added a primal sense of power to Jeremy's outrage. Shocked, he realized the rage he felt might actually cause him to crush the man's skull.

The intruder held his knife at waist level, point extended. The knife's movement followed the baseball bat, the two weapons like cobra and mongoose in their dance of death. The shadowy man began to step sideways.

"Don't move," Jeremy threatened. "Stay where you are." His heart hammered, pumping both fear and rage to every part of his body.

The man took a single step to the middle of the bed and jumped across it. In an instant, he threw open the apartment door and fled into the night.

Jeremy ran after him, whirling the bat round and round over his head. The man veered past the fountain and Jeremy let the bat go when it swung in that direction. "Stop!" he yelled. The bat thudded into the side of the fountain. "Henry, wake up—help me! Somebody stop that man!"

The intruder ran toward the gate. For the first time since jumping out of bed Jeremy realized he was naked. Henry Valadon's lights came on upstairs and his face appeared at the window. "My God, Jeremy, what are you doing?"

Flustered, Jeremy rushed back into the apartment, grabbed a short robe from the open closet and threw it on. When he returned to the patio he heard Henry running down the stairs. "He's getting away," Jeremy yelled, racing toward the gate.

"Who's getting away?" Henry asked. "What's going on? I heard you yell. I saw you running around down here. Are you okay?"

"Some guy broke into my apartment! When I woke up he was right next to my bed. Help me catch him, Henry, he's getting away!"

Jeremy ran ahead and rushed into the street. There was no one in sight. The dark street was quiet—not even a footstep. Jeremy ran to the corner. Still nothing—the man had vanished. Feral cats prowled the Quarter's late-night streets, now drying after the deluge. The only sign of human life was the sweet stench of wet garbage drifting into the air from cans in their sidewalk wells.

Heading back to the apartment, Jeremy remembered Senator Randall's warning. Real danger, he'd said. Could this be the kind of danger he was talking about? How in God's name could some two-bit burglar have anything to do with the rest of it?

Henry was waiting when Jeremy reached the gate. "Did you see anything? Could you tell which way he ran?"

"No, dammit," Jeremy said. "He got away. I should've gone after him buck naked."

Henry glanced at Jeremy's short robe and raised his eyebrows. "I thought you were naked when I looked out the window. What's going on? Who was that guy—somebody you know?"

"Somebody I know? What the hell do you think I was doing?"

Henry shrugged. "I don't know. Some people like rough trade."

"Rough trade? Come on, Henry. I never saw that bastard before. Come in the apartment. Help me check the place out."

They inspected the entry gate and the door to Jeremy's apartment, but found no sign of forced entry. Inside, nothing had been stolen. Jeremy folded the kitchen door fully open and made coffee while he told Henry about the intruder.

Henry smoothed his mustache. "The guy must have planned a robbery—why else would he be here? You probably surprised him when you woke up."

"How do you think he got in?"

Henry shrugged. "No damage to the door—he must've had a key." He walked to the door and turned the knob. "He'd need a key for the gate, too, wouldn't he?" He examined the edge of the door again, from top to bottom. "Hey, look at this. There's a muddy foot print on your rug. The shoe size will be a good lead for the police."

"Police?" Jeremy hesitated. "I don't want to call the police, Henry."

"What? That guy broke in here and assaulted you with a deadly weapon. You have to call the police."

"Why? I probably got that mud on the rug when I ran in here during the rainstorm. No harm's been done except the hole in my mattress." Jeremy glanced toward the bed and saw the distinct print of a muddy shoe in the middle of the sheet, a print about the same size as the one on the rug. Wait a minute…he'd been barefooted when he ran in out of the rain. The senator's words echoed in his head: No one must know of your involvement. "Why can't I just change the locks, Henry? I'll pay for it."

"That's crazy, Jeremy. Insurance will pay for the locks, but we need to make a police report."

The rich aroma of freshly brewed coffee filled the small apartment as Jeremy poured two cups. "Sorry, Henry, no police. I can't tell you why. Not yet. I know it sounds crazy, but I'm asking you to believe me. I'm gonna be working with the FBI and I'd rather not involve the local police."

"FBI? I don't understand."

Jeremy put his hand on Henry's shoulder and looked him square in the eye. "Trust me on this one, Henry. I'll explain later. When you hear the whole story you'll agree with what I'm doing."

"Well...." Henry shook his head and scratched the day-old stubble on his jaw. "Well, okay, since there's no property damage. Still...we don't know how he got the keys—he may be able to get in the other apartments."

"I don't think so. I think it's my apartment, and only my apartment. Just give me time to sort it all out. Try to get somebody to change the locks tomorrow, and let me have the bill."

Jeremy carried his cup to the desk and sat down. He felt certain he'd seen the last of the would-be burglar, but he had not satisfied Henry's concerns. That's what he needed, some way to make Henry stop worrying without betraying the senator's confidence. How in the hell could he do both? How?

41

JOE'S BAD NIGHT

"CAR WRECKS ARE A DIME A DOZEN IN NEW ORLE'NS WHEN it rains." Joe heard his father's words as clearly as if he were standing right beside him. When Joe was growing up Nick Monteleone had said those words every time it rained. He'd always told Joe the rainwater floated oil up out of the black-top and made it slippery. Maybe Papa was right, Joe thought. Charity's Emergency Room had sure been packed since the rain started. An unbelievable number of auto accidents, fender benders mostly, had produced a rash of relatively minor injuries which kept Joe and his team hopping. Few of the patients had serious injuries, but evaluating all of them was tedious business, and Joe didn't get to the sleeping room until after two AM. He locked the door and undressed quickly, exhausted after the twenty-hour work day he'd finally finished.

As usual, Joe fell asleep almost immediately. A short while later he awoke, and that was not usual. He could see it was still dark outside the windows. What's going on, he wondered. He always slept like a rock, never woke up without a really loud alarm clock or the clanging phone. Especially since he got HIV.

He rolled over on his side and saw at once what had awakened him. Squinting through the darkness he spotted a shadowy figure kneeling near the room's door. Damn, it looked like a man—a man wearing a hospital coat. The shadows made it look like he was creeping toward the bed, hunched over, almost like he was crawling.

What time was it anyway? Was it Jeremy, coming in early? Why was he down on the floor like that? He sat up and said, "Jeremy, is that you?"

The dark silhouette stopped moving and stood upright. Damn…it was a man.

"You're not Jeremy—who in the hell are you? What do you want?"

The man stood perfectly still for a long moment, then turned, suddenly, and opened the door. When he ran from the room Joe saw a brief flash, a reflection of light from something in the man's hand. What the fuck...the guy was carrying a needle and syringe. It took Joe a couple of seconds to realize exactly what was going on. This was not somebody's prank. Who in the hell is that guy? How did he get in here?

"Stop!" Joe yelled. He jumped from the bed and ran down the hall after the man. "Come back! Help! Somebody stop him!"

Three or four doors opened into the hallway, and several sleepy house officers in various stages of undress peered out at Joe running down the hall.

The intruder turned the corner and headed down another corridor toward the elevators. He was wearing a hospital coat, but he kept his face averted so Joe never got a good look at him. The man's dark hair was about all Joe could make out. He was average height and weight, clean shaven, wearing sneakers.

Several residents ran into the hallway. One of them grabbed Joe around the shoulders and stopped him. "Take it easy, Joe. Take it easy. What's the matter?"

"That man was in my room. Help me catch him. He's gettin' away."

Following Joe, they all raced toward the elevators, but the fleeing man was nowhere in sight. No one was visible but, just as they turned the corner, Joe heard the stairway door click shut.

One of the residents said, "There's nobody here, Joe."

Another door opened and a tousled head poked out. "Cut out the goddamn noise. You guys have any idea what time it is? Who can sleep with all this shit goin' on?"

Joe ran to the stairway, threw the door open, and raced inside. The stairwell was empty, but on a floor somewhere below, a door slammed.

Baffled, Joe returned to the hall and headed toward his room. The whole floor was in turmoil now, the others began to joke about Joe chasing men down the hall. His bright red bikini briefs, all he was wearing, did not improve the situation. He became a natural target for their teasing.

Sandra Thompson, an anesthesiology resident, opened her door. "What the hell? Oh, sorry, Joe." She did not join the rowdy group in the hallway.

A woman was all it took to incite the floor comedians. A fat OB resident from Mississippi wearing boxer shorts and one limp sock struck a pose in the middle of the hallway. Shaking his curly brown hair, he swiveled his hips and spoke in a falsetto voice. "Oooo-ee, Jo-Jo, take it off. Get nekkid, baby. Sandy likes it, show it to her."

Dr. Thompson closed her door without comment.

"Where'd you get that G-string?" the OB asked.

"I saw one just like it at the Hollywood Shop," someone said. "But that one had sequins."

"Yeah, get some sequins, Jo-Jo. Put gold sequins on it."

"They'll look good in the spotlight, honey. Put 'em on your crotch."

"Come on, Joe-baby. Encore."

They began to clap in unison. "More. More. Take it off—take it all off."

Flushed from all the excitement, Joe tried to laugh it off. He shook his head and walked away. "Come on, guys, leave it alone. Go back to bed."

Once in his room, Joe searched the closet and the adjoining bathroom, but found nothing out of the ordinary. He locked the door to the hallway and propped a chair under the knob. The idea of somebody breaking in the room was pretty farfetched, he realized. He wondered what Jeremy would think when he told him about it. He might not believe it really happened—just like those clowns in the hall.

Joe couldn't think of anything reasonable to do about the break in—not in the middle of the night. But he had made up his mind about one thing. He was not going back to sleep.

With all the lights on, he settled into bed and reached for a pile of surgical journals which he and Jeremy had marked to read. Frightened by the intruder and frustrated by the other residents, he quickly discovered he couldn't concentrate on the dry medical reports.

He wondered how the guy got in. What was he up to? That syringe in his hand...what was he gonna do with that?

Joe scratched his neck and, with a will of their own, his fingers moved to the swellings he'd found there earlier. Damn lymph nodes. He was sorry he'd discovered the fuckers—could mean the worst.

He got out of bed and stretched his neck in front of the dresser mirror. Still nothing visible, and that was good. He'd hoped they might be getting smaller by this time, but they weren't.

He pushed his red briefs down and checked the lymph nodes in his groin. Those were no bigger either. Stable, at least, better than enlarging.

Joe examined every other part of his body where lymph nodes might be found—behind his knees, around his elbows, in his armpits. Shitty luck, he thought. He didn't feel sick, but he was damn glad his quarterly check-up was scheduled in a couple of days. At least then he'd learn how bad it was. Maybe—please, God, let it be—just maybe his T-cell count was still normal Maybe there'd even be some news about a new treatment protocol.

He climbed into bed again, but the long day and the frightening night had taken their toll. Without warning he began to sob uncontrollably. His shoulders shook again and again. Hoarse words poured uninvited from his throat. "Damn, damn, dammit all." He turned over and pounded his fists into the pillow one after the other. "I don't want to have AIDS," he moaned. "I'm not ready to die. Not yet. Please, God, not yet."

42

An Unexpected Twist

Early the next morning Jeremy stopped at a Starbucks near the hospital for two carry-out grandé lattes, then arrived earlier than usual at his fourteenth floor sleeping room. He'd planned his arrival to allow enough time to tell Joe about his meeting with the senator—and now he sure wanted to talk to him about the break-in at the apartment. Unfortunately, he discovered balancing the paper bag of coffee cups and his overnight kit made it clumsy to turn his key in the lock. He could not get the door open.

He put everything down on the floor and tried the key again. The lock worked okay, but the door wouldn't open. Stuck for some reason—he couldn't budge the damn thing. What was going on? It was too early to bang on the door—not cool to wake up everybody on the floor. He tapped on the door with his fingers and whispered, "Joe, wake up. Come on, Joe, it's Jeremy. Let me in."

He was about ready to give up when he heard a scraping sound from inside the room. Then the door opened and Joe stood there in his bikini briefs, looking sleepy and holding a straight chair in one hand.

Jeremy shook his head, picked up the coffee and walked inside. "Man, you really were out of it, weren't you? Tough night?" He lifted the hot cups from the bag and put them both on the desk. "What's with that chair? Did you barricade the door or something?"

Joe shrugged. "I didn't mean to fall asleep. It's been a weird fucking night."

"Weird? Let me tell you about weird. You're not gonna believe what happened to me last night. Sit down—I want to tell you all about it." He crumpled the bag and waved toward the desk. "One of those coffees is for you."

They opened the cups and the early-morning aroma of dark-roasted Columbian swirled out. Each of them told his story of a middle-of-the-night intruder carrying a weapon, then Jeremy went over the details of his meeting with Senator Randall. He told Joe about the senator's investigation, his warnings of danger.

"Looks like he's right about danger," Joe said, draining his cup. "That guy who broke in here didn't actually try to do anything with that syringe, but it's a damn strange thing for a burglar to carry around."

"Really," Jeremy said. "How did he get in here anyway? Was the door unlocked?"

"No, I always lock it. I got in that habit a couple of years ago when those guys on the fifteenth floor were missing some money."

"Yeah, me too," said Jeremy. He walked to the bathroom and tossed his empty cup in the waste can. "Listen Joe, Henry Valadon and I decided the guy who attacked me in the apartment probably had a set of keys. That's gotta be what happened here, too." He paused, then frowned at Joe. "My key ring was missing yesterday, remember?"

"Yeah, what about it? I thought you'd be using my keys, but I saw 'em on the dresser last night and figured you'd probably found your own."

Jeremy nodded. "I did find 'em. I came up here to get your keys after we talked, then I found my own key ring right there on the dresser. At the time I thought I'd had a senior moment or something—thought I just didn't see 'em before. But maybe they really were missing. Somebody else might've had my keys long enough to make imprints."

"Would they've had enough time? When did you last use the keys before that?"

"Well...I rushed up here. I was running late and I unlocked the door—yes, the door was locked when I got here and I used the keys. I took a shower and called Barbara, then I got dressed. I honestly don't remember whether I threw the keys on the dresser or left them in the lock, but I couldn't find 'em anywhere when I was ready to leave. That's when I went down to the ward to look for you, then I came right back here. Somebody could have had my keys for half an hour, maybe more."

Joe nodded. "Long enough."

"What do you think we should do? Senator Randall warned me not to involve anybody else. I hate to just ignore that—he's really trying to help us."

Joe scratched the dark hair on his chest. "You know these crazy break-ins have got to have something to do with all the patient deaths."

"I agree with you there. It's got to be related—happening to both of us like it did."

Joe turned to the window and gazed out. "You said you talked Henry out of notifying the police about the apartment. The situation's different with me, Jeremy—here in the hospital and all. A lot of other people may be in danger. We really oughta tell somebody about it."

Jeremy sat down at the desk. "I can't disagree with that, Joe. But I can't forget what the senator told me. He doesn't know yet who might be part of this whole business. He specifically asked me not to talk to anybody on the hospital staff."

Face flushed, Joe turned from the window. "Easy for you to say, but I don't like it. Obligation and loyalty to a longtime family friend are one thing, but I don't want to sleep in this room as long as lunatics can waltz in here in the middle of the night. And I'm not going to that apartment and wait around for some guy with a knife."

Jeremy waved toward the door. "Maybe we could just get plant management to change the lock on the room door."

"You know that's not enough. This is no time for the Hardy Boys—we need help, Jeremy."

"Okay, okay. You're right, it's not safe to hush it up, but at least I want to call Senator Randall before we do anything." He glanced at his watch. "It's nearly seven—I'd like to wait another half hour. Have you got an early case?"

"No. The juniors can handle morning rounds. Our first case is at nine."

After a quick breakfast in the staff dining room, they were back on the fourteenth floor before seven-thirty, and Jeremy dialed Senator Randall's home number in Beaumont.

The senator's wife answered. "No, Jeremy, Warren's not here. This is Beth. Can I help you with something?"

"What time did they get in last night? I'm surprised he's up and at 'em so early this morning."

"They didn't get here last night, Jeremy. They're still not here."

❖ ❖ ❖

43

Reinforcements

"NOT THERE?" JEREMY YELLED INTO THE TELEPHONE. "I don't understand, Mrs. Randall. They left New Orleans before midnight. The senator's pilot said something about weather, but they've had plenty of time to get to Beaumont by now."

"Oh, they're all right," the senator's wife said. "I didn't mean to frighten you. Warren called about an hour ago to say they're in Austin."

"Austin? What on earth are they doing up there?" He shrugged and shot Joe a puzzled look.

"Warren said a line of thunderstorms hung around Beaumont just when they were ready to come in, and he wouldn't let the pilot make an instrument approach. Austin was their alternate airport."

"And Austin was clear?"

"He said it was. Behind the front, I guess. They all went to a hotel to get a few hours' sleep. Then Warren decided to take care of some business at the Capitol, so I don't expect them here until late afternoon. I could ask him to call you then."

"That's too late—can't we call him in Austin?" Jeremy scratched his head and glanced at Joe again.

"That's the best I can do, Jeremy. They've already checked out of the hotel, and I have no idea how to reach Warren in Austin."

"I'm sorry, Mrs. Randall. I understand. Listen, if he calls again tell him I need the FBI. He'll know what I mean."

"FBI? What's wrong?"

"I'm not sure, maybe nothing, but I'd appreciate it if you'd give him that message."

After that news Jeremy agreed to go with Joe to the hospital authorities. They decided to tell Charles Hollander about the break-in at

Room 1408, but hold off on the rest of it until Jeremy heard from Senator Randall.

By a eight o'clock Jeremy had talked their way past the education director's flaxen-haired secretary, and Joe had told Hollander about the intruder on the fourteenth floor. Hollander walked around his desk to stand directly in front of Joe and Jeremy. "That's quite a story, Joe. I have to agree with you—it doesn't sound like a stunt your house staff colleagues would come up with. You say the man was wearing a hospital coat?"

"That's right," Joe said, "and he had a syringe in his hand."

"What time did all this happen?"

"Around three-thirty, I think. It was a quarter to four when I got back to the room."

"None of the other residents recognized the man?"

"No...actually, they may not have even seen the guy. He made it to the stairwell in a few seconds, and it took a while before the others figured out what was going on."

Hollander peered over his half-frame glasses. "Then you may be the only person who saw the man, right? Has anything like this ever happened to you before?"

Jeremy could not believe Hollander had asked that question.

Joe looked flabbergasted. "You mean hallucination, Dr. Hollander? Is that what you're suggesting?"

"I'm not suggesting anything, but I think we have to look at that possibility." Hollander returned to his chair and sat down, then picked up a silver letter opener and rubbed its smooth surface with his thumb. "You both know what subtle mental changes HIV can produce. Do you have any signs of progression, Joe? Have you had a T-cell count lately?"

Joe's shoulders slumped. He shook his head and glanced at Jeremy, then looked up at Hollander and said, "My quarterly check-up's tomorrow, sir."

Jeremy was not at all happy with the way the discussion was going. It was time for a different tack. "I believe you can put that theory to rest," he said. "There's something else we haven't told you about."

Hollander sat upright and dropped the letter opener on a stack of papers. "Oh? How far out on the limb were you planning to let me go before you chopped it off?"

"I'm sorry," said Jeremy. "That's my fault. The other thing happened outside the hospital, and I didn't want to bother you with it." He told Hollander about the previous night's break-in at Burgundy Street, but he did not mention his airport meeting with Senator Randall.

Hollander picked up a desk pen and made a few notes on a pad. "You think the two break-ins are related, do you?"

Jeremy glanced at Joe, then said, "Yes sir, we both think so. And it looks like they have something to do with those hospital deaths I told you about the other day."

Hollander raised his eyebrows. "Really? Don't you think that's stretching it a bit?" He drew a line at the end of his notes and put the pen back in its holder. "By the way, I asked all the service chiefs whether they'd had any unexplained deaths. They said no. Your own chief said your patient—what was her name, LeCompte, something like that? Your chief said the department files showed her death was caused by pulmonary embolism and chronic pelvic infection."

Pulmonary embolism? Jeremy was astounded. "Dr. Hollander, Mrs. LeCompte did not have a pulmonary embolus. Somebody must have falsified the report. I was at the autopsy and nothing—"

"That reminds me," Hollander said, fingering his desk calendar. "I haven't heard a thing from Marshall Boudreaux about all of that. I thought he'd have called me by now."

"Listen," Joe said, "can't we finish with the other thing first? I don't feel safe sleeping in this building after last night, Dr. Hollander. Can't you arrange some kind of beefed-up security for us?"

"Yes, I can do that. We'll get your lock changed today, but I think we ought to talk to the administrator about anything more than that. Security reports directly to Lockhart. He can arrange it easier than I can."

Jeremy stood up and stepped closer to the desk. "Do we have to go to Lockhart? I haven't had much luck talking to him about anything."

Hollander opened a desk drawer and pulled out a schedule of administrative meetings. "I know what you mean, but I think we need him on this one. Let me set it up, and I'll do the talking. But I do want both of you there in case he has questions." He glanced at his watch then studied the schedule. "Right now looks like the best time to catch Lockhart—before he gets tied up."

"Fine with me," said Jeremy. "How's your time, Joe? You've got a case."

"It'll be close. I might be late—better call the OR."

When they arrived at Lockhart's office Angelina Faget, his secretary, greeted them. "I'm sorry, doctors. He's booked solid until three this afternoon. I won't be able to get you in before that."

"This is important, Angie," said Hollander. "Something he needs to know about."

She shrugged and glanced at her telephone. "He's on the phone right now. I'll ask him when he's finished. But I'll be glad to put you down at three for as much time as you need."

Hollander shoved both hands into the pockets of his hospital coat. "It can't wait until three o'clock, Angie. These men have busy schedules. We're keeping them from their work right now."

Jeremy saw the only lighted line on the woman's desk phone go dark. She must have noticed it, too, because she got up and headed for Lockhart's office. "I'll tell him you're here, but he won't be happy."

A few minutes later, finally inside the office, Hollander closed the door behind them. Lockhart sat at his huge desk, telephone in hand. At the sound of the door latch he stood up, still holding the receiver. "To what do I owe this interruption, Charles? Didn't Ms. Faget tell you I'm busy?"

"She told us. I apologize for forcing our way in here, but something happened last night that I think you need to know about."

"Couldn't it have waited until—"

"No, Larry, I don't think it should wait. Someone got into Dr. Monteleone's room on the fourteenth floor last night while he was sleeping. He woke up and chased the man down the stairs. Joe will tell you the details, but first I want to say I think the intruder definitely meant to harm him."

Lockhart hung up the telephone and walked around the desk. "It must have been some kind of prank." He looked at Joe and Jeremy. "You men work so hard—I don't have to tell you what chronic fatigue can do to a person."

Hollander slashed the air with his open hand. "Dammit, Larry, I told you I think the man intended to do harm. It was not a prank. Just sit down for a minute and hear what Joe has to say. We need your help."

Without further objection, Lockhart returned to his chair. After hearing Joe's story he straightened his tie, then looked at Hollander. "It does sound odd, Charles, but I don't know why you think the man was dangerous. Sounds like he frightened pretty easily." With an overzealous shrug he added, "After all he just ran away." He turned toward Jeremy. "You've been mighty quiet, Becker. What does this have to do with you?"

"Joe and I are roommates, Mr. Lockhart." Jeremy made a quick decision to tell him the rest of it—to put an end to his doubtful questioning. "I was off duty last night, and I spent the night at our apartment. Somebody broke in there, too. He tried to stab me."

"Stab you!" Lockhart waved to Hollander. "My God, Charles, what's going on? Do we have some Jack-the-Ripper chasing after our residents?"

Jeremy grinned at Joe and winked.

"I wouldn't go that far," Hollander said, "but it is worrisome isn't it?" He glanced at the residents, then stood up and moved closer to Lockhart's desk. "These men asked me about added security in the hospital, and I agree with them. It's needed. Can't we do something to tighten things up until we get to the bottom of this?"

"Of course, we can tighten up security in the hospital. I presume the police are involved in the other thing."

Oops, Jeremy thought. Got to keep Lockhart out of that. He said, "It's being investigated."

Lockhart nodded. "Good. Now, about hospital security. There are several things we could—"

The telephone buzzed. Lockhart scowled and picked it up. "What is it now, Angie?" He listened to her reply, then said, "Why didn't the operator just page him?" He listened again, for a longer time. "Urgent? Oh, all right, I'll give him the number."

He jotted a number on a memo pad and hung up the phone. "Becker, there's a urgent call for you—someone outside the hospital. Dr. Hollander's secretary heard your page and told the operator you were here. Angie got the caller's number."

Jeremy took the paper and looked at it. "I don't recognize this number. May I use your phone to check it out."

Lockhart motioned Jeremy around the desk, into his own chair, then joined the others and they talked in hushed tones.

Jeremy couldn't believe it—a day to remember. Lockhart was so polite. Almost human. He guessed they'd made the man happy with a real administrative problem like the security business.

He dialed the number Lockhart had written. After two rings a crusty, low-pitched voice answered. "District Office, Callaghan speaking."

"This is Jeremy Becker. I got an urgent message to call this number."

"Dr. Becker. I'm glad ya called right away. This is Mike Callaghan. I'm Special Agent in Charge of the New Orle'ns FBI district."

Jeremy looked at the others, all involved in a quiet conversation. He could turn away, but it'd be impossible to avoid being overheard. "I'd rather call you back in a short while," he said. "I can't do anything about it right now."

"Can't talk, huh? Good man. Mum's the word, all right. You don't need to talk. Just listen, and I'll tell you what's goin' on."

Jeremy relaxed and leaned back in the chair. "Okay, I'm listening."

Callaghan's throaty voice continued. "Senator Randall called me a little while ago, instructed me to mobilize the team I've had standin' by. Said you knew about it."

"Yes, that's right. What should I do?"

"You don't need to do anything," said Callaghan. "The senator raised the whole business to federal jurisdiction when he got Washington involved. He told me just now to call and let you know the plan. Our team'll contact you sometime late this afternoon."

"All right. I'll be at the hospital."

"Good man. They're gonna need your help to do this job right."

"I'll be here," Jeremy said.

"Okay. They'll find you. Agent Borgne's the team leader, Andy Borgne. Best agent I've got."

"Thank you. I appreciate the call."

"Good man. We'll get to the bottom of it. Senator Randall's been good to the Bureau—we're glad to help 'im out."

The line went dead. Jeremy didn't know whether to laugh or breathe a sigh of relief. As he hung up the phone his mind searched for a way to end the meeting with Lockhart .

Hollander glanced up. "Everything all right?"

"Yes. It really wasn't urgent. Just some information I've been expecting."

"That's good," Hollander said. "Mr. Lockhart has a suggestion for us."

"Yes," Lockhart said, "and it's a good suggestion, if I do say so. Of course, we'll change the locks on your room, and I think both of you men should stay in the hospital for the next few days. I'll have the Chief of Security tighten up the M-E-P restrictions to Condition Red. He'll notify the police, then if anything else happens we'll ask them to get involved."

Jeremy glanced at Joe, hoping for some reaction, but Joe looked distracted so he turned to Lockhart. "Fill me in on Condition Red. I know it's our maximum alert status and only hospital personnel can get through the M-E-Ps, but what else happens?"

"That's right," Lockhart said. "No one else can enter or leave the building. No visitors, no vendors...." He flashed Jeremy a condescending smile. "And no special entry authorizations for family members. We'll have an armed guard stationed at each M-E-P around the clock."

Joe interrupted Lockhart's preening. "Condition Red might not make any difference. It had to be an inside job—somebody who could get the key to our room. Couldn't we just have some guards on the sleeping floors?"

Jeremy tried to telegraph Joe with an intense stare, but he couldn't tell whether the message got through. "We don't really need floor guards, Joe. The whole security system'll be on alert." He glanced at his watch. "Listen, I have to go. I'm about to be late for my staff rounds." He stood and walked toward the door. "Thanks for your time, Mr. Lockhart. We appreciate your help, Dr. Hollander. Thank you very much. We'll stay in close touch about all of this." He opened the door to the reception room, then smiled and looked at Joe. "You going up? I'll get us an elevator."

Joe caught up with him in the hospital lobby and together they walked into an empty elevator. Jeremy glanced sideways at his roommate and pressed the button for the fourteenth floor.

"Okay, Jeremy, what are you up to?" Joe asked. "Your team doesn't have staff rounds today."

Jeremy broke into a grin, then laughed out loud. "Good man."

The mood was contagious and Joe smiled, though he looked confused. "What's going on?"

Jeremy told him about the call from Callaghan and his promise of an FBI team by the end of the day. "We're bound to be safe with the FBI here. Maybe we can finally make some sense out of the whole mess."

Jeremy remained elated throughout his busy day. In the late afternoon, he and Joe met in Room 1408. Jeremy had heard nothing from Special Agent Borgne, and he was getting anxious. "Maybe I should call Senator Randall again. He ought to be back in Beaumont by now."

"Let's wait 'til eight o'clock," Joe said. "Then if—"

A knock on the door startled them both. Each looked at the other with a puzzled expression. Jeremy walked over and opened the door.

An attractive young woman wearing a beige business suit stood there. A large backpack lay on the floor beside her. She smiled and said, "Dr. Jeremy Becker?"

Jeremy stood in the door, dumbfounded. Finally he nodded and said, "Yes."

The woman held up a small leather wallet with an official-looking gold colored badge. "I'm Special Agent Andrea Borgne of the FBI. May I come in?"

44

Andrea

JEREMY AND JOE LOOKED AT EACH OTHER WITHOUT SPEAKING. Jeremy stepped away from the door and watched Andrea Borgne's graceful movements as she hoisted her heavy-looking backpack, carried it across the room, and dropped it in the corner. She was alone. Even if he'd known the FBI might send a woman, Jeremy would never have expected her to look like Agent Borgne.

She was all woman. A conservative, agency look could not hide her soft figure or the laughter in her green eyes. Even if it had, that bright smile was a giveaway—pure femininity. Her honey-brown hair looked long, though it was pinned up and barely cleared the jacket of her suit. A pale yellow, oxford blouse with rounded collars and brown leather shoes with medium heels completed her no-nonsense outfit. On one lapel she wore a circular gold pin with a free-form jade inlay, a whimsical shape of green jade that matched her eyes. Her ears, pierced Jeremy thought, sported smaller circles of the same gold and green design. Something about the way she moved gave hint that a renegade lived inside her.

Finally, amusement showing in his eyes, Joe spoke up. "We expected a team."

Jeremy nodded. "We did not expect a woman."

Andrea smiled and looked at Jeremy. "No one ever does, but don't worry about it. I promise you won't know the difference when we're finished."

"How many of you will there be?" Jeremy asked.

"Two of us here. My partner's Matthew Labordeaux. He got hung up at the M-E-P, but he'll be along soon." She looked from Jeremy to Joe. "Your Condition Red made it difficult to get in here. I'd have been here an hour ago myself, but...." She shrugged. "It's not important—all in a day's work."

"What can two of you do?" Jeremy asked. "This is a big place."

Her eyes sparkling, Andrea laughed. "We only have to cover the inside." She opened her backpack, extended the antenna of a small portable telephone and pressed a button on its dial. "That'll signal the bureau that I'm in place. May I plug in my charger over here? This is the heart of our communications net while we're here."

Jeremy nodded. "I thought you could intercept those things with a scanner."

"Doesn't matter, our phone's too smart for that. It's on a scrambled bandwidth through our satellite. Anything it sends is encoded in a random sequence that changes every half hour. When it receives, it decodes, and what we hear sounds like normal voice."

"You have your own satellite?" Joe asked.

"The bureau has its own frequencies and codes, but we share the satellite with the CIA. Geostationary." She patted the phone and pushed it into the charger. "We have four agents outside the hospital. This baby'll give us secure communication with the others at all times."

Jeremy frowned. "Four outside? That means you and your partner will stay inside?"

"Sure does. Our base of operations needs to be right here."

"Here? In this room?"

She nodded slowly, a twinkle in her eyes.

Joe laughed, but Jeremy was not amused. "Well...I don't know. There're only two beds, and...."

"Don't worry about it," Andrea said. She pulled a large green roll from her backpack. "We have sleeping bags. All we need's a little space on the floor."

"Still, it seems like...."

"Relax, Dr. Becker. Can you do that? You've been up-tight since I walked in here—just relax. I grew up in Terrebonne Parish with five brothers." Her green eyes traveled the length of Jeremy's body then locked on his face. "I don't believe you guys have anything I don't already know about." She turned and walked toward Joe with her hand extended. "You must be Joe Monteleone. Call me Andy." She glanced over her shoulder and grinned. "You, too, Jeremy."

Jeremy smiled and gave her a thumbs-up signal. This was a crazy deal. Barbara was already upset about the gay bar—wait 'til she learned about this arrangement.

Matthew Labordeaux arrived a short time later. He was a trim, brown-haired man, about Jeremy's age, with dark eyes and a short, military style haircut. His handsome face was evenly tanned, but Jeremy was distracted by the large strawberry birthmark in front of the man's left ear, a red, splotchy thing that looked like an oversized paint splatter. Jeremy wondered if it extended into his ear canal.

After Matt shook hands with Jeremy and Joe, he turned to Andrea. "I had a hell of a time getting through that M-E-P. Had to get Callaghan involved."

"Sorry about that," Jeremy said. "It's probably our fault." He told them about the previous night's break-ins. Labordeaux pulled a notebook from his pocket and wrote rapidly while he listened.

"We thought we needed help," Jeremy said. "I couldn't reach Senator Randall this morning, so we told the hospital administrator about the break-ins."

Matt flipped the pages of his notebook. "That's...uh, Mr. Lockhart, right? Laurence Lockhart?"

Jeremy nodded. "Joe and I were in his office when Callaghan called. It was Lockhart's idea to tighten up the M-E-P procedures."

Andrea turned her bedroll on end and sat on it. "We'll have to get our outside men to put a tail on Lockhart. Who else knows we're here?"

"He doesn't know you're here, nobody does," said Jeremy. "We talked to Lockhart and the head of Education, but—"

"Hollander?" Matt asked, looking up from his notebook. "Dr. Charles Hollander?"

"Right." Jeremy turned back toward Andrea. "We told 'em both about the break-ins, but they don't know the senator's involved. And they sure don't know you two are here."

Andrea looked at Matt. They both laughed then, speaking at the same time, said, "Good man."

The two agents had mastered Callaghan's rough inflection, and Jeremy laughed with them. Joe looked puzzled, then relieved. The four of them worked out the sleeping arrangements and agreed on two drawers in the chest for the agents' equipment and the few pieces of clothing they'd brought along.

Senator Randall had faxed copies of his aide's notes to Callaghan, so the agents were familiar with the circumstances surrounding the deaths in the hospital. Matt leafed through the file he'd brought and stopped at one of its pages then turned to Andrea. "You don't really think Lockhart and Hollander are involved in this do you?"

She shook her head. "No, but you know what Callaghan always says."

Matthew nodded, "Yeah." He deepened his voice and gave another good imitation of their boss. "Whatever's goin' on over there, it's prob'ly somebody you'd never suspect."

"He's right about that," Andy said. She looked at the residents and smiled. "We've got Becker and Monteleone staked out, but we'll have to put somebody else on Hollander and Lockhart."

Jeremy looked at Joe and raised his eyebrows. He hesitated, then said, "My...uh, my girlfriend knows about most of this stuff. She went to my meeting with the senator."

Matthew flipped through his file. "That's Barbara Allison?"

"Right," Jeremy said. He shrugged and shook his head. "You guys are way ahead of the game. I'm impressed."

Andrea nodded. "We try." She reached over her shoulder and squeezed the muscles at the back of her neck. "Tell me about Barbara. I understand she's a nurse."

"That's right," Jeremy said. "She's charge nurse on cardiology. Some of the patients who died have been on her ward."

"Will she help us?"

"Sure. She'll do anything she can." Good, he thought. Involving Barbara now might make it easier to tell her about his new roommates.

Andrea got up from the green bedroll, walked across the room and stood facing the others. "Let me tell you the plan," she said. "I want to set up quiet surveillance on some of the hospital wards. We'll need hospital clothing for Matt and me. You two will have to help us pass as visiting residents. You know, teach us the lingo, show us where to go and what to do. We need to disappear into the hospital routine so we can see everything that's happening on the wards without being noticed."

Joe shook his head. "That'll be hard to do, Andy. The other residents'll know something's up."

"You're right, they will," Jeremy said. "I'm not sure we can pull it off."

Andrea looked at them with a wily smile. "You guys underestimate the Bureau. How do you think we got in here anyway? Neither one of us is HIV-positive." She held up an authentic looking M-E-P card with the overprinted outline of a red cross containing the letters N.O.C.H. and the word HIV-Positive.

"Where'd you get that? Looks like a hospital employee card."

"Don't worry about it. We got them—and we're here. Now listen up. Matthew and I will stick with one of you most of the time. You can introduce us as visiting residents from Johns Hopkins—we've got a few more fake credentials. Hopkins ID cards, things like that. With your help we can pull it off, but you can't leave us alone with the other residents.

One or two wrong answers and they'll defrock us." She flashed her green eyes from Jeremy to Joe, then back. "Will you help us do it?"

Jeremy chewed on the lining of his cheek, then looked at his roommate. "What do you think, Joe? Can we make the others believe it?"

"Well..." Joe said, "I think we can probably get it by the other residents. If we're careful. But what about the staff? Even the chief residents would be a problem."

Matt stood up. He pulled a crumpled handkerchief out of his hip pocket and wiped his forehead. "That's a good point. They'd know about any visiting residents, wouldn't they?"

Both Joe and Jeremy nodded.

Andrea waved her hand between them. "Don't worry about that. We can work around it—we'll just stay out of sight when anybody senior to you two is around. We may want to do some surveillance on our own anyway, after you show us around a little bit."

Finally they all agreed they could carry out the charade with a reasonable chance of success. "Okay," Andrea said, looking at her watch. "We'll need most of the night to learn all the right moves, so let's get started."

Matt stopped her. "Wait a minute," he said. "Don't you think we should dust the door to this room for prints? Whoever came in here last night must've touched the knob. The door frame, too."

She began to nod while he was speaking. "Good idea, Matt. Will you do it now? Too bad we can't use the citric acid-gold technique. Better prints." She looked at Jeremy. "Give him a hospital coat, and one of you stand watch in the hall. If anybody comes along before he's finished you'll have to cover for him.

Looking official in a long white coat, Matt managed to collect finger prints from the outside of the door and clean off the black powder before anyone spotted him. "Just give me another couple of minutes," he said. "I want to get these prints in the mail drop to Callaghan before you start the surgery lessons."

"Maybe we should go downstairs for supper," Jeremy said. "I'm getting hungry and we may be in for a long night."

Andrea raised her eyebrows to Matt. He shook his head, and Andy said, "I don't think either one of us feels ready for the staff dining room, Jeremy. Can you order a pizza or something?"

"Yeah. I can do that. There's a place that'll deliver to the M-E-P. We'll have to pick it up down there."

Matt, still wearing his hospital coat, went to the first floor lobby to mail the finger prints. Jeremy ordered two large pizzas, then looked at his watch. "While we're waiting I'd like to call Barbara. Let her know what's going on."

"Good idea," Andrea said. "Ask her to meet us for breakfast. I'm gonna need her help on the cardiology ward." She handed Jeremy her portable telephone. "Here, use this one. No use risking internal wire taps."

Jeremy glanced uneasily at the instrument's unfamiliar dial.

"Just dial Auto-1," Andy said. "That'll put you in the Bureau switchboard. Then it's 8-7 for a city dial tone on a secure line."

Jeremy told Barbara about the previous night's intruders and his need to stay in the hospital for the next few days. He described the arrival of the FBI agents and their scheme to pose as residents. He did not mention the agents' gender. Barbara agreed to meet them in the staff dining room at six-thirty for breakfast.

Matt returned, and all four of them began the challenging task of turning the two detectives into believable surgeons. Andrea and Matt memorized enough hospital jargon to get through most conversations, and they studied sketches of the wards' physical layouts. They listened to detailed accounts of operations the teams performed frequently, and learned what to look for during post-anesthesia recovery. They tried on stethoscopes and otoscopes, tested pen lights and tongue blades, and learned how and when to use them. They wrote down names and descriptions of Joe and Jeremy's team members and the nurses on their wards, and they practiced standing around patients' beds and talking to each other about medical things.

The agents proved to be masters of the deception business, and several hours later Joe and Jeremy agreed they were ready. By that time the room reeked of tomato sauce and pepperoni, and the group was disheveled. An open box of half-eaten pizza sprawled on Joe's bed, and a folded empty was stuffed into the waste can. There was very little time left for sleep before they all worked their way through a discrete rotation of showers and dressing for a new day.

Andrea and Matt put on fresh hospital coats over their street clothes—Joe told them that's what visitors would wear. She unbuttoned her blouse at the collar to show a single strand of pearls, then moved her gold and green pin to the lapel of her white coat.

All four of the odd group looked reasonably authentic as they walked into the dining room a few minutes before six-thirty. "There's Barbara," Jeremy said, waving to a round table near one side of the room. Barbara's body stiffened when she spotted them, and Jeremy decided he'd better talk to her while Joe and the FBI agents went through the serving line.

"Good morning," Barbara said, as he pulled out the chair next to her. Her cold voice reminded Jeremy of a long-ago time he'd been stranded on a frigid ski lift. There was no sparkle in her eyes.

He sat down and angled his chair toward her. "Listen, Barbara, I'm sorry I didn't tell you about Andy last night. There was no reason not to tell you—I just thought it'd be better for you to meet her in person. I didn't know she was going to be a woman until they got here."

Barbara took a swallow from a large glass of orange juice. "It's pretty clear to me she's quite a woman. She's called Andy, is she?"

Jeremy searched for her eyes. "Andrea," he said. "Give her a chance, Barb. She's all business. I know you'll like her when you get used to the idea."

She put her glass down hard, then glanced at Jeremy. Her eyes filled with tears. "Jeremy, this feels like things I wanted to forget about. I've told you how Scottie acted when we were married." She sighed and looked at him again. "You're the only man I've really cared about since that time."

Jeremy touched her hand. "Hey, get rid of those ideas. This is nothing like that." He glanced up. "Look, here they come. Just give her a chance, okay?" He looked into her eyes and smiled. "You're my girl, Barbara. Andy's no competition for you."

He introduced the agents as doctors when they arrived, and he noticed Barbara's quick squint when she spotted Matthew's birthmark. Andrea chose a seat next to Barbara. As Jeremy left the table to get his own breakfast, he heard Joe began a harmless conversation that explained their presence as visiting surgery residents—an explanation he knew was intended for eavesdroppers at nearby tables.

The food servers ran out of grits, and Jeremy waited for more to come out from the kitchen. By the time he returned to the table Barbara and Andy were engaged in friendly conversation. Barbara still acted wary, but she was no longer hostile. Before they finished breakfast she'd agreed to trade shifts and work several nights in order to help Andrea set up surveillance on the cardiology ward.

❖❖❖

45

The Prey

THE FBI AGENTS MADE IT THROUGH EARLY MORNING WARD rounds with no major problems, Matthew with Jeremy's team, Andrea with Joe. Afterward both residents left for their weekly staff conference and the detectives went to Room 1408.

Joe spent the afternoon in the medical library. Jeremy's team was on call and he stayed busy with emergency cases most of the day. When he finally got to the room around six o'clock, both of the agents were sound asleep. They'd been working—papers from their files were scattered all over Joe's bed.

The agents' response to Jeremy's arrival blew his mind. As soon as he opened the door they both leapt out of their sleeping bags. They stood upright with their legs spread apart and both arms extended in front of them. Their two pistols were aimed directly at Jeremy. Reflex made him raise his hands. "Whoa, guys! Hold on. I'm not ready to go through this every time I come in my room."

Both agents looked sheepish and put their guns away. "Sorry about that," Andrea said. "We're trained to do it automatically. It's like a natural defense. Don't forget, at least one stranger has a key to this room. They didn't change the locks yet, did they?"

"Not yet, but I don't care, Andy. I can't go through that every time I come in here. I'm not used to being around guns and I don't like them aimed at me. I can tell you Joe won't like it either."

"Nobody likes it," Matthew said, handing Jeremy a three by five index card. "Here's a coded sequence of knocks I've worked out for all of us to use as a signal before we open the door. That way there won't be any surprises."

When Joe joined the group, the agents described their plan for the night. "Barbara won't be on nights until Monday," Andrea said, "so we'll start on the surgical wards tonight."

"Look, I'm not on call tonight," Joe said. "I have early rounds with my team in the morning, and I need to get some sleep. Last night wiped me out."

Matt said, "That's fine, Joe." Both of you can sleep after you get us set up."

Andrea looked from Joe to Jeremy. "That's right. You don't have to stay with us. We just need you to take us to the wards after the eleven o'clock shift change. Introduce us to the charge nurse, let the patients see us talking, stuff like that. We'll do the rest."

Both residents looked skeptical. "What're you gonna do?" Jeremy asked.

"Don't worry about it," Andrea said. "We probably won't do anything. We just want to see what happens on the wards in the middle of the night. We figured out a way to do that without being noticed, if you'll help us set it up."

Shortly after eleven Andrea left with Joe, and Jeremy took Matt to his team's ward. The ward staff had finished their shift-change report, and Jeremy caught up with the nurse at a patient's bedside. "Mrs. Parrish," he said, "I want you to meet Dr. Labordeaux. He's visiting from Johns Hopkins, and he'll be doing some work on the ward tonight." Jeremy smiled at the patient. "This is Ms. Laura Johnston, Matthew. Laura had a mediastinal cyst removed a few days ago." He noticed the young woman eyeing the red birthmark on Matthew's face. "Chest surgery's not her favorite thing, but she's about to get well in spite of it."

Matt shook hands with Mrs. Parrish and nodded to the patient. "I'm glad to meet both of you." He drew the nurse aside, but spoke loud enough for her patient to hear. "We're doing some work at Hopkins that's related to your HIV research. I need to review the charts of your patients enrolled in the test protocols. I'll record their initial responses to any medications you give them during the night. TPR and blood pressure, any side effects—things like that."

Mrs. Parrish looked at Jeremy. He nodded to reassure her and said, "Matt'll be doing the same thing on the other shifts, but he wants to start with nights."

"That's fine," she said, looking at Matt. "We're used to visitors around here. Just let me know if I can help you, doctor." She turned to Jeremy. "Why don't you show him where we keep the charts while I finish my rounds."

"Thanks, Mrs. Parrish," Matt said with a boyish grin. "I'll try to stay out of your way. By the way, I'd appreciate it if you'd call me Matt, okay?"

Parrish beamed and patted his shoulder. "Don't worry about that, Doctor. Just let me know if you need anything."

Jeremy left Matthew on the ward and returned to Room 1408. He and Joe were sleeping soundly when the phone rang. Jeremy fumbled for the lamp between the beds and turned it on then looked at his watch. Two-fifteen. Neither agent was in the room. He picked up the telephone and said, "Doctor Becker."

"Jeremy, it's Matthew. I need you on the ward."

"What's happening, Matt? What's going on?"

"I'm not sure, but it doesn't look right to me. I need your help."

"Tell me what's happening."

"I can't talk. Just come down here. I'm in the treatment room."

When Jeremy got to the ward everything appeared normal. He stopped at the nurse's desk. "Hello, Parrish," he said. "Everything quiet?"

"Too quiet, Dr. Becker. It's spooky—like the lull before a storm."

"I sure hope not," he said.

The woman chuckled. "I do, too." She looked through the glass partition toward the ward. "The patients are all sound asleep. I don't like it when the ward's this quiet. Listen…you can hear the wind blowing around the building." She looked at a large clock on the wall. "I haven't seen your visitor for a while. He told me he'd be back after the four AM meds."

"Okay, Parrish. I'll find him. You have a good night—don't let the quiet get you down."

Jeremy walked around a corner and down the hall to the treatment room. No light was visible beneath the door. A loud sound echoed from the treatment room, like a bedpan falling to the floor. Jeremy opened the door slowly and went inside. The dark room was filled with the stench of soiled bandages. A man's whisper broke the silence. "Dr. Becker?"

"Yes. Matt, is that you?" Jeremy flipped a light switch near the door. The floor was littered with dirty gauze and bloody tape from an overturned trash can. Agent Labordeaux was crouched behind a soiled linen hamper with his gun drawn, aimed directly at Jeremy. His strawberry birthmark looked even redder than usual.

"What the hell?" Jeremy said. "What are you doing, Matt?"

Labordeaux put his gun away. He stepped out of his hiding place and turned the light off. "Keep it dark, Jeremy. He might come back."

"Who might come back? What are you talking about?"

Matt cracked the door and peered out. He stood near Jeremy and spoke to him in a whisper. "There was a guy out there. Caucasian male, medium height, dark hair. White pants and shirt. Carrying some kind of tray. He went to each of the patients on HIV protocols. He had a flashlight. I couldn't see what he was doing, but he spent two or three minutes at each bedside."

Jeremy peered into the dimly lighted ward. "When did you see him?"

"Just before I called you from that wall phone. I could see him from here. Then he went right past the door and I lost him."

"You didn't see where he went?"

"No. I heard you coming and thought it was him." He turned on the pen light Jeremy'd given him and flashed it around the room. "That's when I kicked over that goddam garbage can."

Jeremy stifled a laugh. "No one's on the ward now, Matt. Let's get out of here."

The two of them walked past the desk where Mrs. Parrish was still charting. "Good night, Dr. Becker," she said. "I see you found your visitor."

Matthew said, "Thanks for your help, Parrish. I'll be back after you give the four o'clock meds to the protocol patients."

Jeremy had a sudden inspiration. "Mrs. Parrish, who's on duty with you tonight. I didn't see a nurse aide on the ward."

"I've got it by myself tonight," the woman said. "My aide called in sick. It looked like a quiet night, so I didn't mind too much." She shrugged and took her glasses off. "Louis Adams from 4B came over here and took the two AM vitals for me. That's what I'm charting now—there's nothing else going on."

"Nice of 4B to give you a hand," Jeremy said. "Adams, you say? Is he an aide on 4B?"

"Yes, he is." She replaced her glasses and picked up her pen. "He's a quiet young man—good aide. It'd help him if you'd write a note of appreciation to the nursing service. You know, helping on the other wards and all that."

"Good idea. I'll do that. Well, goodnight, Parrish." He looked at Matt and slapped him on the shoulder. "Matthew, let's go get a cup of coffee."

The two men left the ward and Jeremy led the way down the darkened hallway to Ward 4B. They saw a black-haired man go into that ward's utility room. Jeremy motioned to Matt, and they followed the man into the small room. "Are you Adams?" Jeremy asked.

"Sure am, Dr. Becker. Can I help you?"

"Do you have any two-inch adhesive tape? My ward's out of it."

"I think we do—let me have a look.." Adams walked to a large metal cupboard and turned the door handle.

Jeremy saw Matthew touch his gun through his hospital coat and begin to move the coat aside. He touched Matt's elbow, then moved his head slightly and squinted. Louis Adams handed Jeremy a roll of tape. "Just leave it on the other ward when you're finished," he said. "We'll restock both of 'em in the morning."

"Thanks, Adams. Goodnight."

When they reached the hallway again, Jeremy stopped and said, "Is that the man you saw?"

"You bet. That's him, all right."

"Okay." Jeremy shook his head. "Let's go get Andrea. We need to have a talk."

They stopped at Joe's ward and asked Andy to join them for coffee in the surgeons' lounge. The three took an elevator to the twelfth floor and found the lounge deserted. A steel coffee urn on a service counter at one side of the room broadcast the aroma of overcooked brew. The shiny pot and their three steaming cups gave the dimly lighted place an air of mystery and intrigue, something like those late-night coffee shops in old-fashioned train stations. Jeremy stood facing the two agents. "Listen, guys, your plan is not going to work." He paused. "You can't learn everything in a few days."

Andrea and Matt exchanged puzzled glances.

"Matt, I forgot to tell you one little thing, one detail, and I thought you were gonna shoot somebody." Jeremy kept his eyes on the man as he spoke. "All the patients on HIV protocols have their pulse and temperature recorded every four hours—including two AM. That's what Louis Adams was doing on the ward when you saw him."

"Okay," Matthew said. "Now we know about it. What's the problem?"

"When I turned on the lights in that treatment room you pulled your gun." He looked at Andrea. "You can't run around the hospital waving guns at everybody that comes along. Either a patient or somebody on the hospital staff is gonna get shot. We have to find some other way to do this."

The two men took a seat. Andrea walked to the coffee pot and refilled her cup. "You're right, Jeremy. We don't know enough about the hospital routines to do it by ourselves. Somebody could get hurt." She frowned. "We might even end up embarrassing the Bureau." She sat next to Matt and glanced at him. "I have another plan."

Jeremy rinsed his empty cup and put it in the sink, then shook his head. "Let's hear it."

Andrea pursed her lips and blew on the hot liquid in her own cup. "We need to set up a trap for whoever's getting to your patients. Leak the word that some patient's a real good candidate for the newest experimental treatment. Then watch the patient like a hawk until whoever it is does whatever he does."

Jeremy shook his head again. "That's no good. Too risky for the patient."

"We can stop the guy before he does anything." She hesitated. "You and Joe will have to watch with us to make sure we don't mess up on some hospital routine."

"I can't agree to that, Andy. Joe and I work pretty hard. We can't do it if we have to stay awake all night with you two." He leaned forward in the chair and extended his arms. "Anyway, you'd still have to use your guns to stop the guy. I won't single out a patient to take that risk."

"Damn it, Jeremy," she said. "We've got to have some reliable way to get to the bottom of all this. If we don't keep it under cover we'll scare the perp away."

Jeremy took a new cup and filled it half way with coffee, then added two splashes of Coffee-Mate. "I have a better idea," he said, looking at the two agents. He stirred slowly, methodically, then returned to his chair. "Let's set up a trap, like you said, Andy. We can leak information about the patient, uh…information about the bait, then see what happens."

Andrea and Matt looked at each other. Both of them raised their eyebrows and Matt shrugged. "I don't understand," Andrea said. "That's what I suggested."

"Here's the difference." Jeremy grew excited. He scratched his jaw, then got up and began to pace around. "We'll use fake information. Fake information about a fake patient."

He stopped and looked at the others, but saw no glimmer of understanding. "I will pose as the patient," he said. "I'll bait the trap, and we'll catch the bastard red-handed."

46

Preparation

THE NEXT DAY WAS A QUIET SUNDAY. AFTER MORNING ROUNDS with their teams, Jeremy and Joe met Barbara and the two FBI agents for lunch. Barbara would be a necessary player if Jeremy's idea for a trap had any hope of success. He knew that might be a problem. She was already a little unhappy about the agents and their sleeping arrangement, and Jeremy wasn't sure she'd agree to take on the role he had in mind for her. Fretting over the best way to persuade her, he decided on a direct approach.

"Barbara," he said when they'd all brought their lunch trays to a table in the staff dining room, "have you arranged to take the late night shift tomorrow?"

"Sure, that was no problem—I make out the schedule." She turned to Andrea. "Do you want to come to my ward tomorrow night?"

"Uh, Barbara," Andrea said, "I think Jeremy has a new plan,".

Grateful for that icebreaker, Jeremy said, "That's right, Barb. And there's no way we can make it work without your help. You'll be a key player in the whole thing."

"Key player…I'm not so sure about that. Tell me about your plan."

Jeremy looked around and lowered his voice. "I'm going to pose as a patient, and I want to do it on your ward tomorrow night. I need your help to pull it off."

"What…? What on earth are you talking about Jeremy? How can you pose as a patient?"

"I've got it all figured out. I'll send Admitting a notice of a planned admission to your ward for a fictitious patient named Joel Lindquist." He looked to Andrea, then back to Barbara and continued his story "Lindquist's coming in for an elective cardiac catheterization to check out the possibility of some kind of congenital heart disease—he's had a bout of congestive failure recently and it's time for a definitive diagnosis. He has to be HIV-positive, of course, and we'll list him as a prime volunteer candidate for testing one of the new protocols from the Research Facility." He grinned. "You can tuck Mr. Lindquist in bed on your ward at the beginning of your shift, then we'll see what happens during the late night hours."

Barbara frowned, then glared at Jeremy. "You've got the whole thing worked out, haven't you? There's only one problem with your silly plan, Jeremy."

"What do you mean? What's wrong with it?"

"The problem is…I don't like it. Not one bit."

"Why not, Barb? What don't you like about it?"

"It's too dangerous, that's what. You know all those patients died. I might as well take you out to the zoo and feed you to the tigers."

Andrea laughed. "I hear you, but you don't have to worry about his safety. Matt and I'll both be close by—we'll make damn sure he's safe the whole time. We'll be ready for anything that comes up, anything at all." Matthew nodded and flashed a grin so big it wrinkled the birthmark near his left ear.

Joe's left hand touched his own neck. "Wait just a minute, everybody. What's my role in this crazy scheme? Why can't I be the fake patient—then Jeremy can help the two of you keep me safe. How does that sound to you, Barbara?"

Jeremy said, "That won't work, Joe. You're on call tomorrow night, remember? Suppose our patient, Joel Lindquist, has to jump out of bed in the middle of the night and run down to the ER."

"Come on, Jere. You could take my call."

"No," Jeremy said. "It's settled. I'm going to bait the trap. We'll see who we catch—we'll find out who'll take the bait, or try to take it."

After another half-hour's back and forth discussion about Jeremy's plan they all agreed to go along with it. Barbara was still reluctant, but she finally agreed. Jeremy pulled an admitting slip from his coat pocket, an admitting slip he'd already filled out for a patient named Joel Lindquist. "I'll drop this off at the Admitting Office right after lunch."

Barbara shook her head. "Jeremy. You already worked out every little detail, didn't you? What if I hadn't agreed to your plan?"

Jeremy blew her a kiss. While he went to Admitting, the others headed to the house staff gym on the sixteenth floor. The gym had been converted into a cinema while all the residents were staying in the hospital full time. Someone had a collection of Laser Disc movies and they were showing a film version of one of Tennessee Williams' plays in the makeshift movie house. Andrea had concealed her portable phone in the pocket of her borrowed hospital coat and warned Jeremy to call her if he had any problem before he joined them on the sixteenth floor. "Call me about any trouble," she said. "Anything at all."

He had no trouble. His admitting slip included all the needed information about Mr. Joel Lindquist and his scheduled admission to the cardiology ward on Monday evening. The staff parking garage was within the hospital's security zone, and Jeremy needed some clean shirts he'd left in the Miata the day before the M-E-P lockdown started. He decided to stop by the garage before heading up to the movie.

The garage was dark when he got there, but he remembered where he'd parked so that was not much of a problem. Feeling his way through the dim space, Jeremy noticed a beam of light flickering around the parked cars—not moving in any purposeful way, just flashing around helter-skelter.

What the hell? Looks like somebody's walking around with a flashlight. Maybe a security guard checking on the cars. Weird, that's not something they'd normally do. Better check it out.

He moved closer to his Miata, and the light grew brighter, more focused. Who was that? A tall, lanky man wearing a jacket and tie—damn, looks like Mr. Lockhart. Why the hell would the administrator be skulking around the parking garage like that? Whoa, it was Lockhart and he was shining his flashlight all around the rear deck of the Miata.

Jeremy stepped out of the shadows. "Mr. Lockhart. What in the world are you doing in the garage? Can I help you?"

The light flashed to Jeremy's face. "Becker," Lockhart said. "You startled me, creeping up in the dark like that."

"I'm the one who should be startled, Mr. Lockhart. Why are you looking around my car? Is something wrong?"

"I hope not, Becker. Is this your car? Well…the chief nurse told me she thought she had a flat tire, and I'm trying to check it out for her. She said her car was a small sports model—I thought this might be it. I'm just checking the license plate."

"Well, this is not the car you're looking for. Maybe I can help you find it—what's the nurse's license plate number?"

Lockhart fumbled in his jacket pocket for a moment, then said, "Oh, don't bother, Becker. I don't want to keep you from your work. Thanks anyway."

Jeremy opened the Miata's small luggage compartment and picked up an armload of clean shirts on hangers. Lockhart wandered away in the dark garage, flashing his light here and there.

After putting away the clean shirts in Room 1408, Jeremy joined the others on the sixteenth floor. The film had already started and he had to squeeze past several others to get to the chair Barbara had held for him. "Sorry, guys…excuse me…sorry about that." An anesthesia resident stood to let Jeremy pass and her chair overturned with a loud clatter.

Finally the confusion settled down, but Jeremy could not follow the movie's action. His mind was spinning over that business with Lockhart in the garage. What was he up to? What was all that BS about a flat tire? Lockhart didn't even know the plate number of the car he said he was looking for. What would he do, anyway, if he found the damn car? Change the flat tire himself? Not likely, not Lockhart.

After the movie they all decided to take it easy for the rest of the afternoon. Everyone was keyed up in anticipation of their plan for a trap on the cardiology ward the following night. Andrea updated Jeremy and Joe about the agents working outside the hospital. She said Agent Raintree and Agent Rizzo were tag-teaming surveillance of Dr. Daniel Hebert from the HIV lab. Others from the Bureau were tailing Laurence Lockhart as well as Dr. Charles Hollander, but none of those agents had fake M-E-P cards, so their surveillance was only outside the hospital.

That news surprised Jeremy. He didn't realize they were already watching Lockhart. He told the others about running into the administrator in the staff garage and his weird story about looking for a car with a flat tire. "Andrea, maybe you should change Lockhart's surveillance to include inside the hospital. He's crazy and unpredictable—no way to know what he'll do next."

Barbara had left the group soon after the movie, saying she had some chores at home. Andrea and Matt wanted to scope out the cardiology ward and finalize their plans for close oversight of the next night's trap.

During the evening Jeremy had a half dozen calls to the Emergency Room to advise his junior residents about managing minor injuries, but it turned out to be one of those unusual nights when none of the injured patients needed urgent surgery. Even so, he didn't get too much sleep—he knew the next night would be difficult. Like an unfamiliar operation he was about to perform, he kept running through every possibility for trouble while he posed as a patient to bait the trap—kept working out solutions for unforeseen problems. He stayed awake long into the night repeating a mental what-if analysis, reviewing and re-reviewing every detail of their plan to ensnare a killer with him as bait in the trap.

❖ ❖ ❖

47

A Clandestine Meeting

While Jeremy was scurrying to and from Charity's Emergency Room, Special Agent Bruce Raintree sat in his unmarked sedan parked in view of the garage exit from Dr. Charles Hollander's condo. It was an older building, slightly run-down, but the garage had only one way in and out, so Raintree's job was easy. He lighted another Camel and turned up the radio volume to better hear the soft music from station WWL.

Raintree was a bear of a man—a large American Indian who'd chosen law enforcement after he graduated from law school. He was convinced no law firm would take on a guy like him, and he knew he'd never make a living in independent practice. Tribal life on the reservation was not for him—leave that to those lazy guys he grew up with.

A few minutes before six-thirty a car drove out of the condo garage. That was his man—Raintree knew the car, a gray older model Chrysler. He threw his Camel out the window and followed a half block behind the Chrysler, close enough to keep him in sight but far enough to escape notice. Wonder where he was going this time?

After a roundabout cross-town drive, he watched as Dr. Hollander parked on Magazine Street, close to a place with a big sign above the door that read, Casamento's Restaurant. Raintree knew Casamento's was one of those long-established small restaurants, slightly out of the way on Magazine Street—not actually in the Garden District, but close. He'd never been there, but he'd heard the place had some of the best seafood in the city. Okay, if Dr. Hollander wanted seafood, he was willing.

He watched the doctor walk into Casamento's, then parked his own sedan a half-block away. Inside the restaurant he managed to sit at a table across from Hollander—near enough to see who joined him and hopefully to overhear some of their conversation.

He heard Hollander order a glass of white wine, then saw him look impatiently at his watch. Fifteen minutes later Hollander was still alone, and he ordered another glass of wine. Before the second wine arrived, the restaurant's door flew open and a tall middle-aged man waltzed in with a flourish like he owned the place—a stocky guy with graying hair, he wore an expensive looking charcoal gray double-breasted suit. The newcomer glanced around the room, then headed toward Hollander's table. He and the fresh glass of wine arrived at the same time.

Hollander thanked the waiter then stood to greet his dinner companion. "Good evening, Mr. Boudreaux. I'd just about given up on you."

"Dr. Hollander," the new guy said, "Well, I did ask you to meet me here. I would never stand you up—not an important man like you, Director of Education and all."

Both men sat down. Agent Raintree pulled a small notebook from his jacket pocket and discovered the name, Boudreaux, on the list Andrea had faxed to him: member of the hospital's Board of Trustees, chairman of the HIV Lab's Finance Committee. Damn, this must be some kind of high powered meeting—those two. Why would they choose this place way over here on Magazine? Why not meet at the hospital?

Raintree kept one eye and an ear on the other men's table while Boudreaux ordered a full bottle of the same wine Dr. Hollander was drinking, along with a twelve-inch oyster po'boy with extra oysters, no ketchup. Hollander chose a large bowl of seafood gumbo, and they told the waiter they'd share a dozen oysters on the shell. Hollander said, "Bring extra horseradish for the oysters, if you will."

Raintree knew it wouldn't be easy to pick up the men's conversation, but he turned on his pocket recorder just in case. He had ordered a smaller oyster po'boy himself, and iced tea to drink. If those two stayed long enough, he might have dessert afterward—pecan pie or something like that. The Agency was paying. Damn, he wanted a smoke, but he knew he'd have to wait. Straining to hear the men over the hubbub of the popular restaurant, he heard only bits and pieces, just enough to get the gist of what their meeting was all about:

"The names of all the residents in the surgery program…."

"What on earth…?"

The waiter rattled Boudreaux's wine bottle noisily into a cooler of ice. The conversation continued:

"Believe me, I can make it worth your while."

"...a brand new Chrysler?"

"That's nothing. What about a seven figure retirement fund?"

"...list of every patient who volunteers for the HIV Lab's test protocols."

"...confidential...."

"Come on, we're both insiders...."

"Starting when?"

"Tomorrow. Can you do that?"

Their dialogue continued along those lines throughout dinner. Raintree made enough notes to jog his memory later when he wrote his report for Andrea.

Boudreaux and Dr. Hollander seemed to reach some kind of agreement. Halfway through Raintree's pecan pie they both left Casamento's together, joking and laughing their way to the door. Mr. Boudreaux had picked up their bill. He had also pulled a fat leather case that looked like an overstuffed wallet out of his breast pocket and passed it to Dr. Hollander.

Raintree called for his own bill and paid it in cash to get out of the restaurant as quickly as possible. He reached his sedan just in time to see Dr. Hollander's Chrysler pull away from the curb. He followed Hollander as long as he could, but lost him when he turned into the staff garage at Charity Hospital. Damn, Raintree's HIV-negative card would not allow him to go through the M-E-P at the garage entrance. He'd told Andrea all along he needed a fake HIV card if he was supposed to tail anybody on the hospital staff. Oh well, next time. He lighted a Camel and called her on his secure phone to report that Dr. Hollander had entered the hospital. He'd pick him up later when he left the building.

❖ ❖ ❖

48

THE PREDATOR

JEREMY AWOKE AT DAWN TO FIND ANDREA SITTING ON HER ROLLED-up sleeping bag, busy in conversation on her secure portable phone. He was on the way to the bathroom when she ended her phone call and put the instrument away. "Morning, Jeremy. Ready for the big day?"

Jeremy raised his eyebrows. "Big day? Oh, yeah, the trap. I'm about as ready as I'll ever be. But right now I have a major case in the OR, and I have to get going."

"Okay. I do have a few things to tell you about when you finish your shower. It won't take long—if you're having breakfast I could go down there with you."

After his shower and shave Jeremy found Joe and Matthew also awake. "Hey, Joe, why are you up so early? You don't have a case this morning, do you?"

"No, but I've turned into a light sleeper in the last few weeks. I thought I heard you and Andrea talking, then the sound of your shower woke me up completely. He smiled. "I dreamed it was pouring rain outside."

Andrea said, "Matt and I figured out a pretty good hiding place on the cardiology ward for tonight's trap. We're ready to keep you safe, Jeremy, and, with any luck at all, we'll take our perpetrator in custody at the same time—whoever that is."

"What else is new?" Jeremy asked. "I saw you talking on your phone."

"Right. Special Agent Tony Rizzo has been tailing your administrator, Mr. Lockhart. So far he's clean as a whistle. He lives alone in an apartment in the City Park area. Nice neighborhood. Rizzo called it mid-middle class. Lockhart went to a symphony performance last night, then straight home afterward. Nothing he's done is suspicious in any way."

"What about all that weird stuff in the garage yesterday? Hanging around my car and all that?"

"That was probably innocent, Jeremy. I found out the chief nurse really did have a flat tire, and her car looked something like yours. She did ask Lockhart to check it out for her, and he arranged to get a Triple-A repair guy in the garage to change the tire."

"I don't get it. Lockhart told me no visitors could get through the M-E-P during Security Condition Red."

"Well, he is the administrator—he must have found a way to work around that restriction. Anyway, the whole thing looks legit to me."

"Whatever," Jeremy said. "Just keep your tail on Lockhart. I still don't trust him. Any other news from the outside agents?"

"Nothing important. I'm waiting for a full report from Bruce Raintree, but he left a message saying Dr. Hollander drove into the hospital parking lot around nine-thirty last night. We may have to get a fake HIV card for Raintree so he can watch Hollander when he's in the hospital. Our agent following that Hebert guy from the HIV lab told me he stayed home last night—watched some TV, read a research journal, and went to bed early. He did have one phone call later, but the wiretap wasn't working right so we couldn't tell who it was."

"Okay, thanks for the update. What are you and Matthew planning for today?"

"I've got a little telephone business with Callaghan at the office," Andrea said. "I want to talk him into getting a fake HIV card for both Raintree and Rizzo. And, Matt, I want you to hang around Dr. Hollander all morning. Buddy up to his secretary—try to figure out what he's doing in his office, who he talks to on the phone, things like that. This afternoon we should both try to get some sleep. We probably have a long night ahead of us."

"Well, let's all meet for supper in the staff dining room ," Jeremy said. "I'll call Barbara and ask her to join us. Is six-thirty okay with your schedule, Joe?"

"Should be fine," Joe said. "I have staff rounds this afternoon, but that won't take too long. If I'm lucky I may even get to take a nap. I've been feeling a little under the weather lately."

Both residents had their usual busy day. Joe did manage time for a late afternoon nap before he and Jeremy met the FBI agents in the dining room at six-thirty. When they'd all brought their food trays to an empty table in a corner of the room Andrea asked, "Is Barbara coming, Jeremy?"

"No. I spoke to her around noon and she said she'd just see us on her ward after eleven tonight. She wanted to get some rest before her late shift."

Joe said, "Andy, did you and Matt learn anything new today?"

"Nothing from me," Andrea said. "I did manage to get a fake HIV card for Raintree so he can stay on top of Hollander. Callaghan wouldn't go for two of 'em, but Raintree's okay. I'm still waiting for his full report about whatever Hollander did last night."

"Why are you paying so much attention to Dr. Hollander?" Jeremy asked. "He's the one person on this hospital's admin staff we can trust completely."

"You never can tell, Jeremy…you just never can tell. Like I told you, Callaghan always says, 'The one you least suspect is probably the one you're after.' What about you, Matt?" she asked. "Did you learn anything new today?"

Matthew flashed that big grin that wrinkled his birthmark. "Well…maybe nothing too important, but I did have a pretty good time trying. Besides being a real cute blonde, that Colleen Shannon is quite a gal."

"Colleen Shannon?" Andrea said. "Who in the hell is Colleen Shannon?"

Jeremy and Joe both laughed. Jeremy said, "What's the matter, Andy? Are you jealous? Colleen is Dr. Hollander's secretary."

"Cut it out, guys," Matthew said. "I did learn a couple of things from Colleen that might be interesting. Dr. Hollander asked her to get him a list of names and addresses for all the surgery residents—told her to print it up so he could give it to one of the Trustees."

"Which Trustee?" Jeremy asked. "Did she say which one?"

"Doesn't matter," Joe said. "That's probably nothing. Hollander is Director of Education."

Jeremy frowned. "Surgery residents only? That includes you and me, Joe. What's that all about, Matt? Did Colleen know why a trustee wanted the list?"

"She didn't say—but there is one more thing. Hollander also asked Colleen to contact the charge nurse of each patient ward and make of list of every patient who's volunteered for the HIV lab's test protocols—names, ages, hospital numbers, all that."

"That sounds odd. Why did he want that?"

"Colleen didn't know why, but she started telephoning around to get the names before I left her office."

Andrea shook her head. "Like I said, Jeremy, you just never can tell…."

After supper, Joe and the agents went to Room 1408. Jeremy went to the ICU to check on the patients his team had operated on earlier in the day. The four met outside Barbara's cardiology ward at twenty past eleven. She'd told them that would give her enough time to finish her shift-change report and say goodnight to the nurses and aides from the earlier shift. Joe went into the ward ahead of the others to be sure none of the earlier shift staff were still around. Jeremy wore casual street clothes instead of his usual hospital garb.

As they hoped, Barbara was alone. She'd assigned the nurse aide some made-up task in the supply room, and she'd dimmed the ward lighting. She hustled Jeremy away from the others before any of the patients had a chance to see his face. "Quick, go in the linen room. I put a full set of patient clothing in there for you. After you change I'll bag up the things you're wearing now. Admitting sent up all the paper work for your late admission as Mr. Joel Lindquist. I'll put you in that corner bed away from the lights."

Jeremy changed into the pajamas and cloth slippers Barbara had left for him, then slipped on a cotton robe to complete his transformation from doctor to patient. Barbara came back into the linen room and attached a pre-printed ID bracelet to Jeremy's left wrist. Carrying a clipboard with Joel Lindquist's admitting information, she showed him to the corner bed she'd selected. She went through the business of recording his initial vital signs and asking about his home medications then, in earshot of the patients in adjacent beds, she said, "Mr. Lindquist, your doctor left admitting orders for you. He said he'd see you real early in the morning since your procedure in the cath lab is an afternoon case. Get some rest now—just press your call button if you need anything at all."

Jeremy looked all around the darkened ward, but saw no sign of a reasonable hiding place for the FBI agents. Damn, he hoped they could see him way over here in this dark corner. Joe was on call, so he'd gone back to Room 1408 to avoid the possibility of his beeper going off during whatever action lay ahead on the cardiology ward.

All of the other patients were quiet, probably sleeping, Jeremy thought. He'd had a long day himself and lying down felt pretty good. The bed wasn't too bad. Firm—no, it was damn hard, but not too uncomfortable for one night. In less than ten minutes he was asleep. Barbara had told the nurse aide not to awaken the new patient for two

AM vital signs.

Jeremy slept soundly until nearly four, then he woke up suddenly with an urgent sense that someone was standing at his bedside. He turned and peered into the darkness. Barbara? No, not Barbara…it was a man. A man wearing a hospital coat and carrying some kind of tray and a flashlight. "Mr. Lindquist?" the man asked.

"Yes, I'm, Joel Lindquist. Why?" The man was dark-haired, medium height, but Jeremy couldn't make out his face. Where in the hell were those FBI agents?

"I'm from the lab—need to draw some blood. Screenin' tests for that HIV protocol you volunteered for." The man put his tray on the bedside table and pulled a rubber tourniquet from it. He took Jeremy's left arm and pushed up his pajama sleeve.

"Hold on a minute." Jeremy said. He pulled his arm away and groped around for the call button—maybe Barbara could stop this crazy man if the agents weren't coming to the rescue. He pressed the button several times in rapid succession. Dammit, what was that Morse code for SOS?

"Just let me have your arm," the dark-haired man said. "This won't take no more than a second." He jiggled his flashlight beam around the bed. When the light moved over Jeremy's face the man drew back from the bed and gasped. "Dr. Becker. Why are you in this bed? Did they hurt you again?"

That voice? Who in the hell…?

At that moment the ward blazed into full light. Matthew and Andrea ran to the bedside, guns at the ready. Barbara was right behind them. The dark-haired man abandoned his tray. He turned away from the bed and headed for the door, but Andrea stopped him. She blocked his escape with her spread-legged shooter's stance, both arms extended, gun aimed directly at the man's chest. Matthew grabbed both his arms and twisted them behind his back. He locked handcuffs around the man's wrists then spun him around facing the bed. Jeremy sat up and stared, dumbfounded. "Leonard Guidry—what the fuck are you doing here? How in the hell did you get all that lab stuff?"

Guidry did not resist. He stood motionless and hung his head in silence. Andrea said, "Leonard Guidry? Is that what you said, Jeremy? That name's on our suspect list."

"Right," Matt said. "And some of the fingerprints from your room door matched a person named Leonard Guidry."

Andrea put the gun in her shoulder holster. "Well, we've got the bastard now. Good job, Jeremy, Are you okay?"

Jeremy sat up and slipped his feet into the cloth slippers. "Oh yeah, I'm fine—what took you guys so long to get over here?" He waved toward the lab tray. "Guidry was just about to go after me with a needle."

"The nurse aide discovered our hiding place at the wrong moment," Andrea said. "No problem…it doesn't matter now. We've got the guy. We'll see you in the morning."

"Where are you going?"

"Don't worry about it. We've got some business to take care of."

The two agents manhandled Guidry out of the ward in handcuffs. Barbara scurried from bed to bed, reassuring all the other patients. Jeremy returned to the linen room to get out of Joel Lindquist's hospital clothing.

When things quieted down, he took Barbara aside. "Thanks for your help, Barb. The trap worked like a charm. There was one thing, though—why didn't you come right away when I hit the call button?"

"Your light never came on, Jere. As you sure you pressed the right button?"

"Damn right I'm sure. Let me show you." They walked to the now-vacant bed. Jeremy picked up the call button and pressed it a few times. Nothing happened. He traced the button's cord to the wall socket and found it unplugged. The connection was broken.

He shrugged. "No wonder—you never even knew I called. For a housekeeper, Guidry's a lot smarter than I thought he was."

Barbara picked up the lab tray. "May as well get rid of this stuff so we can get the bed ready for a real patient. Should I just send it down to the lab."

"That should work." He glanced at the lab tray. "Hang on a minute, Barb. What's that in the tray? It's more than empty syringes and blood collection tubes." He picked up a ten c.c. syringe resting on a small warming pad and attached to a shielded needle. "This syringe's got some kind of cloudy liquid in it. Damn—Guidry must have planned to inject me with whatever this stuff is. Ask the lab to culture it for viruses."

❖❖❖

49

INTERROGATION

"WHERE ARE YOU TAKING ME?" GUIDRY ASKED THE FBI agents.

"Shut up, Lennie, "Andrea said. "We're going to a quiet place where we can talk."

"Those iron things hurt my arms. Can't you take 'em off?"

"Not yet, Lennie. Not yet."

The agents pushed Guidry into an elevator and pressed the button for Basement. On the way down, Andrea pulled a card out of her pocket and read Guidry his Miranda rights. Guidry said he understood. He told her he did not want an attorney. They jostled him at high speed down the dark basement corridors toward the old tunnel that once lead to the medical school across the street. Matthew fished a key out of his pocket and opened the padlock at the tunnel entrance.

They walked in, shoving Lennie ahead, then continued to a small store room at the far end of the tunnel. Matthew used his key again and they all went in the store room, and pushed Guidry into a straight chair next to a small table. Matthew slammed his pistol down on the table.

"How'd you get that key?" Guidry asked. He could see nothing much was left in the store room. "I thought my key was the only one besides that laundry woman."

"Don't worry about the key, Lennie," Matthew said. "I want you to look at this machine on the table. It's a tape recorder. You know what that is don't you?"

Guidry nodded. "Yeah, I know what it is."

"I want you to speak up when you answer our questions so we can get it all on the tape."

Merde, not much of a room they'd brought him to...that table and the chairs, one little mirror on the wall...that was about it, outside of that tape recorder. He'd answer their questions, all right...tell 'em anything they wanted to know. He hadn't set out to hurt anybody like Dr. Becker—not him. Danny told him it was only patients that were gonna die anyway. That part was okay, but not Dr. Becker. Not a nice man like him. He was nowhere close to dyin'.

Andrea switched on the recorder and said, "I'm gonna ask you one more time, then that's it. Do you want a lawyer?"

"No, I told you. No lawyer." *Quelle chierie!* Pain in the ass! The woman had been asking that same question ever since they left the ward. He'd said no from the beginning—why didn't she stop asking?

Andrea walked behind him and unlocked the handcuffs. "Show me your wrists. Do they feel better without the cuffs?"

"Yeah, it's all right now." Good woman. Reminded him a little bit of Mama, wantin' to be sure she didn't hurt him too bad even when she had to be mean. He thought about Danny? Why in the world did Danny trick him like that…trying to get him to shoot that stuff in Dr. Becker's veins. Good thing he found out who it was…just in time, too. Well, that was the last time Danny'd trick him. He'd see.

The interrogation moved ahead. Guidry could tell both agents were bein' soft with him, especially the woman. He answered all their questions real easy. He told 'em how Danny Hebert had set up the whole thing—he was the boss. Danny picked the patients for injections and told Guidry where they were in the hospital.

He told the agents how Danny had taught him to puncture the veins and fixed up the lab tray for him. He'd showed him how to turn on that little warmin' pad he put in the bottom of the tray. Guidry found a good hidin' place for the tray and all that stuff in the tunnel. Danny had always called him beforehand, then brought the syringes to him in the tunnel just before he used 'em.

"Didn't you know your injections would kill the patients?" Andrea asked.

"No. I didn't know that—not at first anyway. Danny didn't tell me that part, but I figured it out after a while. We had a big fight over that, but he told me it was okay. Told me the patients he picked were gonna die anyway."

"You thought that made it all right, did you? Made it all right to kill people because they were going to die anyway?"

"Danny said it did."

"And you believed him?"

"Sure. Danny's real smart. I always had to talk to him when I finished, you know. Tell him exactly what happened."

"Lennie, how long have you known Dan Hebert?"

"A long time...he was about the same age as Weldon. Between Weldon and me."

"Who's Weldon?"

"He was my best friend...he died when he was sixteen. He'd be in his thirties now, if he'd lived. That's when I met Danny—after Weldon died. A grown man told me about Danny."

Andrea stood up and stretched her shoulders, then walked around the table and stood behind Guidry. "Are you tellin' us you and Daniel Hebert grew up together?"

"Not exactly. I grew up in Thibodaux and he lived over in Golden Meadow. He was Weldon's friend more than mine—Weldon and his brother, Raymond. Weldon started coming around our place when he was twelve or thirteen. Mama never did like Weldon, but after I went to Miss Rena's we ran around together all the time."

Matthew adjusted a knob on the tape recorder. "Tell us about Dan Hebert. What was he like when he was a boy?"

He didn't want to talk about that, not yet. "Weldon and me were just about the same age. His daddy always said he was gonna make their whole family famous when he was a priest."

Andrea said, "Lennie, we don't care much about Weldon. Just tell us about Danny. Did you get along okay with Danny?"

Not yet…he had to tell 'em about Weldon first. "Weldon's mama said he could be the pope if he put his mind to it. He was a real good looking guy—all the girls at school ran after him. He played football, too. First string quarterback in his senior year. That's the year he died."

Andrea shook her head and shrugged. "Okay, tell us about Weldon, Lennie? Why did Weldon die?"

Not so fast—she had to hear the whole thing, then maybe she'd understand. "Well, we had this secret place over by the bayou…grown up all around with thick cane, except under that big ol' cypress tree. It was a good swimmin' hole. Nobody else knew about. Just about every day we went swimmin' over there, diving off the cypress knees and all. You know how them knees stick up in the edge of the water?"

Andrea nodded and smiled at Matthew.

"Well, the two of us were jumpin' around buck naked, then I came up from a dive right in front of Weldon. Real close to him. We just stayed like that for a while...then he took me by the hand. We ran out of the water and went in a clearing we'd made in the cane, like a little room with a floor made out of an old quilt. Our clothes were in there, but we didn't put 'em on. We just—"

"Lennie we don't care about that stuff. Just tell us what you and Dan Hebert did?"

"I didn't do nothing with Danny 'til a long time later—it was only Weldon at first. Then Weldon died in the hospital."

"In what hospital, Lennie? Did they bring him up here to Charity?"

"No. He was in the hospital in Thibodaux...the whole thing was my fault."

"What do you mean? What was your fault, Lennie?"

"That's what I'm tryin' to tell you. One day when we was swimmin' I dared him to dive off that cypress limb. Well, naturally, Weldon did it. He climbed up that big tree, naked as the day he was born, and flew right down toward the bayou. I knew them cypress knees were all around where he was gonna hit, but it was too late. He hit one of 'em all right, then he went under the water and didn't come up." A low pitched wail rumbled out of Guidry's throat and tears flooded down his face.

"My God, Lennie. What an awful thing to see."

"In the hospital they found out Weldon was paralyzed from his neck down. He was out cold, never even blinked his eyes. They hooked him up to a breathing machine—said he'd die without it. Three or four weeks later Weldon was still unconscious. It wasn't natural, all them tubes and everything—that machine breathing in and out for him all the time. I felt like he was already dead or somethin'. Maybe God was punishin' him for what we did at the bayou. I couldn't let him stay like that."

"What did you do, Lennie?"

"Like I told you, I couldn't leave my best friend like that, so I kissed him on the forehead and unhooked the breathing machine. He was gonna die anyway. Right then his brother, Raymond, slipped out of the closet and told me he saw what I did. He saw me kill my best friend. He warned me I better always do what he said or he'd tell his mama I killed Weldon. Later on Danny Hebert said Raymond'd told him all about it, so I better do whatever he said, same as Raymond."

"And you believed Dan," Andrea said. "Is that why you injected the hospital patients for him?"

"I did everything for him. Even went in that doctor's room up on the fourteenth floor like he told me to. Danny said the doctor was dyin' of AIDS, and I was supposed to inject him. But it didn't work out like that. The doctor woke up and almost caught me before I ran down the hall."

"Why'd you do it, Guidry? Why did you keep on doing that stuff after all those years?"

"Ray and Danny never let me forget what happened. After I came to

New Orle'ns Danny wrote to me once or twice a month. Never a real letter…he'd just write, 'I know you killed Weldon' or something like that. Kept it up when he went to college—never would let me forget it." Guidry leaned forward, holding his head in both hands. His body convulsed in a seizure of uncontrolled sobbing.

"You probably didn't really kill Weldon, Lennie. Sounds like that dive out of the tree killed him. Why'd you let those two keep you down like that?"

Guidry took a deep breath and let out a long sigh. He stared at the ceiling. "It was that hick town...that and my daddy."

"You grew up in Thibodaux, didn't you say?"

He nodded, but kept his eyes on the ceiling. "We were dirt poor, lived like trash. My daddy didn't care, he was a mean man. The very first thing I remember about him is a beatin'. I couldn't have been more than four or five, and he beat the shit out of me. For no reason—said I wasn't payin' attention to things he told me."

"Didn't your mother try to stop him?"

"Mama stop him? Shoot, she was so scared of that man she couldn't stop anything. I always thought he musta beat her from the day they got married. They had one other boy a couple of years older than me—he died around the time I was born."

"So, what did your father have to do with Ray and Danny?"

"I killed my daddy."

"What? When did that happen, Lennie?"

"I killed him when I was eleven. Daddy'd kept on beatin' me, then, when I was nine or ten, the fuckin' started."

"You mean...?"

"I mean he raped me. Kept on doing it. Three or four times a week he took me in the shed—told Mama I needed a whippin', but it weren't no whippin' he was after. Said he'd kill me if I told Mama what he did, and I believed him. A few months after I turned eleven—I was a pretty big boy by then—I went in the shed while he was out on the shrimp boat. I hid a brand new ax handle where I could get it in a hurry."

"A day or two later my daddy took me to the shed. After he finished, he told me to put my clothes back on. I bent over like I was tying my shoes, then I picked up that ax handle and hit him with it. Hit him hard, right in the face. Took him by surprise, I guess…he fell down. He was bleedin' a lot from a big gash on his forehead. I hit him again and he rolled over. He tried to crawl to the door, but I kept on hittin' him with that ax handle until his head was a bloody mess and he didn't move no more. I knew he was dead. I didn't care."

"My god, Lennie, what happened after that?"

"I was real scared 'cause I knew I'd have to talk to the sheriff about it. That sheriff was a big ol', ugly man and I was afraid he was like my daddy. I didn't know what to do, then I figured out how Mama could help me. I ripped my pants and smeared Daddy's blood all over me. I started crying and ran in the house half naked. I told Mama we found a hobo hidin' in the shed. He beat Daddy with the ax handle, I said, then he fucked me and took off toward the bayou."

"Did she believe you?"

"She believed me...I never was sure about that sheriff, though." A smile flitted across his face. "That's when I met Mr. Boudreaux."

"Mr. Boudreaux?" Andrea looked at Matthew. "Are you talkin' about Marshall Boudreaux?"

Guidry nodded. "Yeah, he still came to Thibodaux a lot in those days. The sheriff was his brother-in-law. When Mr. Boudreaux heard what happened, he came to see me. Looked out for me like a big brother. Mama died a couple of years later, and Marshall practically adopted me. Bought all my clothes, gave me money when I needed it, moved me in with his sister—that's Miss Rena. He owned her house, and he stayed there with us when he came to town. Sometimes he took me to New Orle'ns for holidays with him and his wife."

"Did Boudreaux have any children?"

"No. I was like his son, I guess. I learned a lot from talking to him...one day he told me he'd figured out I killed my daddy. They found Daddy with his pants unzipped and his dick hanging out. Mr. Boudreaux told me he'd talked the sheriff out of charging me for killin' Daddy."

"Did you live with Marshall Boudreaux when you came to New Orleans? Do you still live with him, Lennie?"

"Naw, not any more. I lived at his house for a while. Dan Hebert was there a lot, too. When I told Mr. Boudreaux I didn't want to go to college he made me leave. He said I had to make it on my own, but later on he got me this housekeeping job at Charity."

Matthew turned off the tape recorder. "That's enough for right now, Lennie. Listen to me, you are under arrest for attempted murder. We have to take you to over to the Parish Prison tonight. They'll take you to the judge in a day or two. Turn around and hold out your arms."

"You have to put those irons back on me? Can't you leave 'em off? I won't do nothin'."

"I have to put 'em on you, Lennie. Let's go."

❖❖❖

50

Closing the Net

IN SPITE OF JEREMY'S LATE NIGHT AS BAIT IN THE TRAP TO CAPTURE the interloper on the cardiology ward, he was up early the next day for morning rounds with his team. Later, before he finished breakfast in the staff dining room, his beeper rang out. What the...he didn't have a case in the operating room and he didn't expect an ER call so early in the day. He knew Joe was in the operating room, and he hadn't seen either of the FBI agents since they hustled Guidry out of the ward in the middle of the night. Using the wall phone to answer the beeper, he learned his father had telephoned from Beaumont, so he headed to his room for privacy to return the call.

"Hey, Dad. I got your call. What's up?"

"Good morning, Jeremy. Senator Randall telephoned a little while ago with some news he wanted me to pass along to you. His Judiciary Committee concluded their investigation in a late meeting last night. He told me they confirmed all the shenanigans he was worried about."

"Shenanigans? What do you mean, Dad?"

"I mean all that business at your hospital and at the HIV Research Facility."

"I hope it's good news. What did they come up with?"

"Well, it is good news for us. Their investigators uncovered all the sordid details of a long-standing relationship between Marshall Boudreaux and Congressman Pierre Legrande. Those two grew up together in Thibodeaux. Seems like they're lifelong buddies, and when Legrande first ran for Congress, Boudreaux spearheaded his campaign fundraising."

"Sounds pretty normal to me."

"Hold on, Jere. Years later Legrande's seniority in the House of Representatives helped push the Health Protection Act through Congress, and he was in a position to ensure huge appropriations for the HIV Research Facility. You remember all that ultra-high tech stuff we saw over there—Legrande pushed through the money for all of it. Then, after the lab was up and running, he made sure funding for world class research would continue to pour into that facility to the tune of six million dollars a year."

"I like that part, Dad. I'm counting on those guys finding a cure real soon so I can get this damn virus out of my body."

"What's the matter, son? Are you feeling okay? When's your next check-up?"

"I'm fine, Dad, but I'm tired as hell of taking a handful of meds every single day—the meds I take just to keep things under control. You know…not a single one of them offers a real cure."

"Jeremy, consider the alternative."

"I know, I know. But our Research Lab is on the brink of something really promising. There's even buzz about a Nobel Prize, and I want that money to keep pouring into the Lab."

"Okay, Jere, but there's a lot more to it than that—listen to me. In his position as Chairman of the Research Lab's Finance Committee, Marshall Boudreaux has managed to siphon off a big chunk of those appropriated millions. He's manipulated things to get his people in position to control all of the lab's purchasing and procurement. Most of the equipment and supplies, and all the billings for them, flows through dummy corporations Boudreaux owns. He can even control distribution of some of the private research grants. Much of that money will never find a cure for anything. Now listen to the rest of it—you remember what Senator Randall told us about Congressman Legrande's extravagant life style?"

"Right, I remember what he said—boats, planes, vacation houses, foreign travel, all that."

"Yes. Well, it looks like Marshall Boudreaux has been funding, much of Legrande's extravagance. Both of them have been living high on the hog, and Boudreaux provides most of the finances."

"My god, Dad. Do you mean those two are stealing federal funds intended for the HIV Lab? What can the Senator Randall and his Judiciary Committee do about that?"

"Warren told me they're getting the FBI to go after Boudreaux today. And they're sending their report to the House Ethics Committee with a recommendation to impeach Congressman Legrande. No matter how that comes out, Warren's confident Legrande will be indicted for misappropriation of government funds."

Jeremy chuckled. "Sounds like the Thibodeaux gang is folding up. Well, now I have something to tell you—more about the good ol' Cajuns from Thibodeaux. Last night we set up a trap on Barbara's ward and caught—"

The door flew open. Loud laughter burst into the room ahead of Andrea and Matthew. "Oh, sorry, Jeremy. I had no idea you'd be here."

"Dad, can I call you back in a few minutes. My temporary roommates from the FBI just came in, and I need to hear what they've uncovered since last night's trap."

"Make it quick, Jeremy. I have something else to tell you—something important, and I'm busy in the office this morning."

"Okay, Dad. Ten minutes." He hung up the phone. "Andy, Matt, what's going on? What did you do with Guidry last night?"

"Well, our friend, Guidry, told us some surprising stuff," Andrea said. "He's in Orleans Parish Prison right now. He'll be indicted tomorrow morning for attempted murder and probably more. By the way, I'm sure you'll have to testify when he comes to trial."

"I expected that. When will it be?"

"Don't know yet—probably months from now. But there's more, Jeremy, lots more. Matt, tell him what we else learned from Guidry."

"Okay," Matthew said. "It turns out Leonard Guidry was in a long-time affair with Dr. Daniel Hebert from the Research Lab. We believe Hebert's been blackmailing Guidry for most of his adult life."

"Okay…their affair jibes with seeing them together in that bar in the Quarter. But, blackmail—why in the world would Hebert blackmail a guy like Guidry? He's got nothing."

"It's a complicated story, but Guidry thinks he killed his boyfriend when he was a teenager. Hebert learned about it, and he's held it over Guidry's head for years. Guidry told us he killed his own abusive father, too. Remember that Hospital Trustee, Marshall Boudreaux? He's involved in all of this. Fact is, he was probably behind the whole thing."

"Why in god's name would any of those people want to kill our hospital patients?" Jeremy asked. "Why in the hell was he going after me when he thought I was a patient?"

Andrea said, "We don't know that—not yet. But hang on a minute. Here's another news bulletin that's gonna blow your mind. She pulled a few folded sheets of paper from the pocket of her hospital coat. "Here's Agent Raintree's full report about Dr. Hollander. Raintree followed Hollander to a dinner meeting with Marshall Boudreaux at a restaurant on Magazine Street."

Jeremy shrugged.

"Sounds okay, does it? Well, during their dinner Boudreaux asked Dr. Hollander to get those lists Matt learned about from his secretary—the surgery residents' names and all the volunteer patients. Hollander agreed to do it and Boudreaux gave him a pile of money with promises of a lot more in the future."

"Damn it all," Jeremy said. "You can't trust anybody, can you?"

Andrea grinned. "Maybe not, Jeremy, especially when big bucks are involved."

"What about Mr. Lockhart? What have you learned about him?"

"So far, he's clean," Matthew said. "Rizzo's been staying right on him outside the hospital, and I've been snooping around his office. Looks like Lockhart's nothing but an insecure dandy who thinks a little too much of his own importance, and he really enjoys playing up to the Board of Trustees. Nothing we've found links him to any of the other stuff."

Andrea said, "Listen, Jeremy, finish your phone conversation with your father. Matthew and I are heading down to Hollander's office right now to take him in custody for questioning."

"You're going to arrest Dr. Hollander?"

"Well...yes. It'll probably lead to that." Both agents checked their pistols in their shoulder holsters and left the room.

Baffled, Jeremy dialed his father's office number and got him on the line after a short wait. "Dad, it's me again. You had something else to tell me?"

"Yes, Jeremy, it's something important. Maybe the most important thing Warren told me this morning."

"Okay...shoot, then I have some breaking news for you."

"Warren's Judiciary Committee got wind early today of something suspicious going on between Marshall Boudreaux and Charles Hollander. They don't know the details yet, but I want you and Barbara to be very careful around the hospital. I'm not sure you can trust any of those turkeys in charge of the place. Just be careful, Son."

Jeremy laughed. "I hear your warning, but it's a little bit too late, Dad. That's my breaking news. The FBI agents are on the way to Hollander's office right now. They're going to arrest him."

"What? That's a surprise. I suppose it's the things Warren's people learned about, whatever that is."

Jeremy's beeper buzzed again. "I think you're right, Dad. Listen, I have to go now. I'll be in touch later."

"Yes, I heard your beeper. You better see who needs you…and, Jeremy, don't fret about your medications. They're your best hope right now."

The call was from the Emergency Room. Jeremy's whole team was caring for the victims of a relatively minor auto crash, but the sheer number of patients had overwhelmed them. An entire family was involved, two parents, one mother-in-law, and four children. Their car was broadsided at an intersection by a pickup truck jumping the traffic light. Fortunately, none of the family was seriously injured. They all had myriad cuts and bruises that required x-rays and a few stitches, work that kept Jeremy tied up for more than an hour and a half.

When things settled down and he was ready to leave the ER, he saw Andrea standing at the trauma room door. "I have big news to tell," she said. "Can we talk here?"

Jeremy led her to a vacant treatment room and sat down on a roll-about stool. "What's going on now, Andy?"

"Agent Rizzo just called. He was on surveillance today out at Boudreaux's mansion in Metairie. About an hour ago he spotted Boudreaux leaving the house with a bunch of luggage."

"Was his wife with him? Maybe they were going on vacation."

"No, Jeremy, Boudreaux was alone. Rizzo stopped him for a few questions. That might have ended it, but Boudreaux objected. Rizzo told him Congressman Legrande was in trouble and Dr. Hollander had been arrested. He tried to bluff his way out of the whole thing, but Rizzo won—he took Boudreaux in custody for questioning."

"Where did Rizzo take him? Is he in jail?"

"Not yet. He's at our headquarters—Callaghan's interrogating him right now." She grinned. "Just wait 'til Boudreaux hears the taped conversation Raintree recorded on Magazine Street. I don't think he'll need much luggage for the trip he'll take when Callaghan finishes with him."

❖❖❖

51

NOLA Redux

Jeremy and Andrea were heading out of the ER when the ambulance dispatcher rushed up behind them. "Hold on a minute, Dr. Becker. You need to know about a call I just got. The FBI is coming in with somebody from the HIV lab. They said something about NOLA, does that mean anything to you? They used your name—told me to call you."

"Who's the patient? Did they say?"

"They didn't tell me a name."

Jeremy thanked the dispatcher, then checked to make sure a trauma room was available. He wanted a room with a little privacy. Didn't matter who they were bringing in—might be a chance to learn more about what to expect from that NOLA strain.

A few minutes later two aides and a nurse wheeled a gurney in from the ambulance ramp. A large man in civilian clothes was running close behind them.

"What the hell?" Andrea said. "That's Agent Raintree. He was supposed to be following Dr. Hebert."

"Following Daniel Hebert?" Could it be? Yes, by god, it was him—Hebert was on the gurney.

Jeremy waved the ambulance crew into the trauma room and stepped close to help them lift Hebert to the treatment table. While the staff removed Hebert's clothing, Andrea introduced Bruce Raintree. So this is the Indian, Jeremy thought. Giant of a man. "Good job, Raintree. I heard about your work at Dr. Hollander's dinner meeting."

Raintree shook Jeremy's hand. "Thanks. I feel like I already know you, Dr. Becker. Andy and Matt have kept all of us up to date on things going on in the hospital. We've been busy outside, too. Security at the HIV Lab gave me a little trouble, but this morning I managed to get part way inside to keep an eye on this Hebert guy." He gestured toward the patient on the trauma table. "About half an hour ago he staggered out of the lab's maximum security zone and collapsed in the lobby—he couldn't even walk, took two big guys to help him."

The trauma nurse reported, "Blood pressure one-ten over ninety-two, pulse one-oh-eight. His temp is one-oh-one."

"Get an IV going," Jeremy said. "Ringer's lactate. I believe we're dealing with early septic shock. Hook up the monitor, and get ready for an A-line."

Jeremy turned back to Raintree. "Did they tell you what happened to him?"

"Something about an injection. He gave himself some kind of shot."

Dan Hebert raised his head. "No arterial line, okay? It's too late to do much anyway."

Jeremy glared at him. He pulled down the sheet covering Hebert's body and touched his skin. Hot, clammy. Dusky looking. Hebert's eyes were moist and glassy. His pupils were constricted. So, this was the guy behind Leonard Guidry's scheme to kill our patients. The bastard probably doesn't even know Guidry tried to kill me last night.

"What did you do, Dan? What did you inject? Was it the NOLA Strain—did you inject NOLA into your own body?"

Hebert closed his eyes. "It was the only way, Jeremy. Everything was falling apart around me. No way could I spend the rest of my life in prison. I know what NOLA did to those patient volunteers—I knew it would be quick and painless."

"You worthless crock of shit. Not one of those patients chose to die—you took away their chance to live long before AIDS took its toll. And what about the rest of us—all of us whose hopes for a cure were linked to what you could do with NOLA. What about us, Dr. Hebert? What about the millions of us around the world?"

Jeremy knew Hebert was on the brink of serious shock and he felt a primal instinct to do nothing. After all, the guy had injected the damn virus into his own body? He could just walk out, stall for time, let nature take its course. That urge shocked Jeremy—it ran counter to everything he knew, counter to everything he believed in. Hebert might not deserve help, but that was a moot point. Jeremy knew he would do everything he could to keep the man alive.

"What about the A-line?" the nurse asked.

"Hold off for right now. But do start a second IV and put a Foley in his bladder. Better give him some aspirin by rectum, too. Thirteen hundred milligrams." He leaned close to Hebert. "You're in my world now, Dan. It's me, not you, who decides what we do here. If you think I'm gonna let you get away with your little cop-out, forget it. Life is too precious for a bum like you to call the shots."

Agent Raintree moved from the corner of the room and touched Jeremy's arm. "Okay if I record this, Doc?"

Jeremy nodded, and Raintree started the tape in his pocket recorder.

Both IVs were running fast, and one of the aides was checking Hebert's blood pressure every couple of minutes.

"Why?" Jeremy asked Hebert. "Why did you do it?"

Hebert opened his eyes. "What do you mean?"

"Don't give me that bullshit. I know the whole story, and I mean all of it. Why did you hire that two-bit burglar to go after me at my apartment? Why did you set up Guidry to attack my roommate? Why did you kill our patients?"

Hebert glanced away. His wavering gaze wandered around the room and finally came to rest on Jeremy's face. "It's a long story, man."

"Start telling it, you've got nothing but time now. You're not going anywhere—I won't let you get off that easy."

"There's nothing you can do. I took a bigger dose than we gave any of the patients."

"Was it really the NOLA strain?"

Hebert nodded, and his lips separated in a half smile. "It won't take long, not with the amount I injected. Must've been an hour already."

"One-oh-four over ninety. Pulse ninety."

Jeremy noticed there was only a trickle of urine in the collection bag. "Speed up both IVs—run 'em wide open. And give him a double dose of steroids in the IV line."

"No use to bother with any of that," Hebert said. "I know this virus."

"You may know the virus, but I'm not going to let you die before you start talking."

"One-oh-eight over ninety-two. Pulse ninety-four."

Hebert cracked a little smile. "I had a rough time growing up down in the bayou country. My dad was a small town physician, but he was a mean son-of-a-bitch. He beat the shit out of me and my little brother all the time. One day, I finally decided I'd had enough. While he was beatin' me I grabbed him by the neck and choked him 'til he passed out. I knew what happened, but everybody said he had a minor stroke, so I went along with it. He never was the same again. He lived, but he had to give up his practice and all. Marshall Boudreaux found out about it from the sheriff, but nobody else knew I choked him. Then, when Lennie Guidry came over from Thibodeaux I found out his family was even worse. Lennie killed his dad, you know—killed his own boyfriend, too. He was no angel."

"I know all about Lennie. Sounds like a bunch of rotten families, but I can't buy it as a reason to kill people." He glanced at Raintree to be sure the recorder was working. Raintree nodded.

"One-ten over ninety. Pulse ninety-four"

Hebert continued his tale. He rushed on like there was no way to stop talking now that he'd started.

"One-twelve over eighty-eight. Pulse holding."

Hebert gave a weak smirk. "Marshall Boudreaux said he'd take care of me. He took care of me, all right. Look where I ended up."

"He must have helped you when you were a boy."

"Yeah, he did I guess—paid for college, travel, lots of things I could never have done without him. I felt like I owed my whole life to him."

"You said Boudreaux recruited you to come back to New Orleans."

"I told you that?"

"Yes, when I took your lab tour."

A sardonic grin twisted Hebert's face. "It wasn't exactly recruiting. I was happy in D.C., but he wanted me down here—threatened to publicize what I did to my daddy if I didn't agree to it. He'd found out I was gay, too. I didn't really think that would make any difference in my job at NIH, but he said he'd use it against me. Between both things, he really put the squeeze on me."

"Why was he so insistent?"

"Wanted me to do his dirty work. He...." Hebert blinked a couple of times and sighed, then his eyelids closed.

"Ninety-eight over eighty. Pulse one-twenty."

He was breathing rapidly. His skin was paler than before and the sheet covering him was soaked with sweat. He defecated loudly on the table. "Repeat the steroids," Jeremy said. "Run in two units of plasma expander, and get a vasopressor drip ready to go. Keep the other IV wide open."

Hearing a new sound behind him, Jeremy looked over his shoulder and saw Raintree changing the micro-cassette in his recorder. Maybe they've got enough, he thought. Didn't matter, he wanted to hear more. He wanted to know why the whole damn plot had swirled around him—wanted to know whether he was still in danger. He watched the saw-tooth tracing on the EKG monitor as Hebert's heart rate slowed in response to treatment. "Come on, Dan, tell me the rest of it. What happened after you came to New Orleans?"

Hebert struggled to open his eyes. "Nothing happened at first. Then, after a few months, drug testing in the lab was really moving along at high speed, thanks to the NOLA strain. *In vitro* testing of our double drug protocol suggested it would be a real breakthrough treatment for AIDS. There was no sign of animal toxicity and we were ready to begin human testing. That's when Boudreaux got involved."

"One-oh-four over eighty. Pulse one hundred."

"What did Boudreaux do? He should have been glad the lab was doing well. It could have been another feather in his cap."

"Yeah, he should have been glad. But he decided if the protocol was as good as we said, HIV research would go out of business in a year or two—we'd have a cure. If federal funding stopped, he'd go broke. He was draining millions out of the budget in contracts for phony companies he'd set up, and he didn't want anything to change that. He did not want our treatment protocol to succeed, and he decided to make damn sure it didn't."

"How could he stop it? The scientists must have realized how promising it looked."

"That was my job. Boudreaux told me to block the protocol. He'd stolen an enormous amount of money from the lab, and he promised to make it worth my while. He didn't care how I sabotaged the protocol. Just don't let it succeed, he ordered. Swore he'd ruin me if I didn't go along with it."

"One-oh-two over eighty-two. Pulse up to one-ten."

"The only thing I could think of," Hebert went on, "was to prevent completion of phase one trials in the volunteer patients. I knew the FDA would never let us test the protocol's effectiveness until we confirmed it had no toxic side effects in humans. I had to be sure none of the volunteers made it through the toxicity trials. To do that, I needed somebody in the hospital, and Boudreaux told me about Leonard Guidry working here."

"You knew Guidry before, didn't you?"

"From Thibodaux and Golden Meadow. I knew he was in New Orleans, but I didn't know what he was doing."

"How did you pull him into your scheme?"

"Ninety-six over eighty. Pulse still climbing, one-sixteen."

Practically no urine flow now, Jeremy noted. "Give him one more dose of steroids. And start the vasopressor. Keep the IVs running fast."

Hebert gave a weak cough and continued. "I knew the NOLA

would do what we had to do. There'd never been a human infection with that strain, and it would take a while before anybody could identify NOLA as the cause of the patient deaths. I'd planned to get rid of the first one or two volunteer patients, then pull the protocol out of testing. That would have delayed things long enough to think of something else while we redesigned the protocol."

"You didn't pull the protocol, Dan. What happened?"

"Too many people got involved. I told the others in the lab we were running into some kind of unexpected toxicity, but patients were clamoring to volunteer for the protocol, and nobody in the lab wanted to pull it out of testing. They said I'd used bad selection criteria, chosen volunteers with advanced disease—pushed me to keep on testing. They thought that would lock in the Nobel prize for the NOLA strain. That's when I tried to limit the volunteers by having all of them go through you. Slow it down, at least, but I lost control of that, too. You and your team were too good at signing up patients. Then Boudreaux got involved again—told me to get you and your roommate out of it. He wanted to get rid of both of you."

"Eighty-eight over seventy. Pulse one-twenty-four."

Jeremy was concerned. Looked like the virus had completely destroyed Hebert's immune system. He was failing in spite of everything. Maybe there was no way to stop it. Maybe his body's normal bacterial flora, now undeterred, might be behaving as invasive pathogens infecting every vital organ, smashing the delicate equilibrium of a near-perfect ecosystem. "Speed up the vasopressor."

"Eighty-four over sixty. Pulse one-thirty. His temp's up to one-o-three."

"Okay, give him another six-fifty milligrams of aspirin, and let's try one more dose of steroids. Keep the vasopressor going."

Hebert sucked in a noisy, gasping breath. "I thought the jig was up when you treated Anderson in the Emergency Room."

"Anderson? Who's that?"

"The man from my lab who came in here after his auto crash. I thought you'd figure out he must have gotten the NOLA strain from that broken pipette and see his death looked the same as the patient volunteers. I really lost control after that...wanted to stop, but Boudreaux wouldn't let me...I had to keep on killing the patients you signed up. I felt like I was on a treadmill and couldn't get off." He looked toward Raintree. "Until that big lug came along...his snooping around got people suspicious and bought the whole thing crashing down."

"Seventy-eight over fifty. Pulse steady."

Moving his head, Hebert motioned Raintree to come closer. "Take it easy on Leonard Guidry, man. He didn't understand any of it. He was just a poor dumb kid who loved his boyfriend too much...loved him way too much."

"What about Guidry?" Jeremy asked. "How'd you talk him into doing your dirty work?"

Hebert's breathing was fast and shallow. His eyes closed.

"Fifty-five over zero. Pulse sixty."

Jeremy watched the steadily slowing rhythm on the EKG monitor until it straight-lined. Shaking his head, he turned to the nurse. "No code, okay? This patient had a terminal illness."

52

Hope

BARBARA SIPPED BLACK COFFEE WHILE READING THE LAST PAGE of Jeremy's draft for his keynote address at the AIDS Conference. The early November air was warm in their Garden District condo. The wake-up smell of cooking bacon wafted from the microwave. She put her empty cup and the manuscript on the table, then removed her reading glasses and smiled at Jeremy. "I really like this, Jere. It's pretty sneaky how you slipped in those comments about the housekeeper and his pal from the HIV Lab without revealing how you discovered they were working as a team."

"Thanks—I guess sneaky is a compliment. I thought their scheme needed to be included in the speech, but after your fussing about Guidry last night I didn't want to mention their names." He kissed her on the forehead. "Marshall Boudreaux ran the show, you know, but those two were his front line operatives in the whole chain of events that led to collapse of the Health Protection Act. They were the key players in everything that happened."

"Are you going to tell the conference about putting yourself on those front lines? Wouldn't they like to hear about the trap you set? Tell 'em how you deliberately put yourself in harm's way as bait for the trap."

"Well…I don't know about that."

"Why not? You may as well be the hero in this piece, Jeremy. What you did was way beyond the call for a surgery resident."

"Yeah, I guess you're right, but that trap also led to some bad things, Barb."

"What do you mean, bad things? You got rid of the crooks—you ended their cruel murders of patients volunteering for the HIV treatment protocols. You triggered everything that brought the whole evil scheme crashing down."

"Right, but we also ended mega-funding for the Regional HIV Labs—completely stopped their work on the HIV-NOLA strain. We put an end to any hope for our lab to win a Nobel Prize, and we probably delayed, maybe delayed for decades, any hope of finding a cure for the damn HIV."

"Come on, Jere…you don't believe all the things Senator Randall uncovered and what he did about them were a waste of time. You know he could never have gotten so much done without uncovering the whole plot right here in New Orleans. Your late-night trap on my ward at Charity made it all happen."

"All right, all right. What you say is true, but cutting out the research funding and ending the Health Protection Act also meant I could never practice surgery the way I wanted to…damn shame Joe's not around to hear my address. He'd be stuck in education, too."

"That is a shame. I miss Joe."

"And don't forget ending the HPA also ended your career in hands-on nursing, Barbara. Once the HIV segregation ended neither one of us could do the things we'd worked toward for our whole lives."

"Doesn't matter. You're doing okay in education. So am I. And the HIV suppressing drugs did get better in spite of all that research funding going away. True, we're both HIV-positive, but we're still pretty healthy. We've had no complications, and our T-cell counts are normal. They can't even identify the virus in our bodies anymore."

"Thank God for all that," Jeremy said. "But teaching residents outside of the operating room is not what I had in mind. And I bet if you had your druthers, you'd be running a busy ward full of patients instead of lecturing nursing students."

"Well, I don't deny that, Jere, but consider the alternative."

Jeremy grinned. "You sound like my dad. It's really hard for me to stay optimistic, you know. Working on this speech has made me think about how close we came—how different things might have been if a few greedy individuals hadn't screwed everything up for us."

She stepped behind his chair and slipped her arms around his shoulders. "Think positive, doctor. Someday a cure will come—maybe we can still do all the things we wanted to do. In the meantime, we have each other, and we enjoy life. We can't give up hope."

"Right, but what we need, Barbara, is a cure. A real cure."

"Listen, you know the researchers are coming up with better and better treatments every year."

"Yeah, some of 'em look promising all right, but it's not yet the cure we need.

"That'll come—just you wait and see."

"We should live so long, Barbara. We should live so long."

A few weeks later, on World AIDS Day, Jeremy stood alone at the podium in the Louisiana Superdome. Some two thousand physicians, scientists, and other interested parties were seated below on the stadium floor. All eyes were focused on the keynote speaker. A pair of latecomers rushed in and found seats near the back row. Jeremy spotted Barbara standing at one side of the crowd. The huge room grew quiet.

"Ladies and gentlemen, welcome to New Orleans. Welcome to the annual World AIDS Conference." He waited while the audience settled. "Today I wish to tell you about a man who wanted to be a surgeon. An unforeseen accident got in the way of his dream. The thing we all fight, the dreaded HIV, interrupted that man's designs. He joined the ranks of the millions of HIV-positive persons around the planet."

Jeremy shifted his weight. Someone in the audience coughed.

"Soon after the man's conversion to seropositive, fear took over—growing fear of an HIV epidemic spreading like a wildfire across this country from sea to shining sea. Politicians shared peoples' fears, and they enacted the Health Protection Act of 1989." Jeremy smiled. "The new kind of segregation required by that law did allow the man I'm telling you about to complete a surgical training program, and that was good.

"Huge appropriations of federal monies led to great promise of a cure for HIV infections. But much of that promise was cut short. Greed entered the picture and dashed those shining hopes. A self-serving scheme carried out by a handful of men sacrificed HIV-positive individuals for their own personal gain, and led to the end of federal largesse for AIDS research. The greed of those few sabotaged the researchers bright promises. It extinguished the flame of hope for a cure that had appeared to be imminent."

Jeremy stepped to the side of the podium and ran his eyes along the front row of his audience.

"In addition to subverting AIDS research, those greedy actions destroyed the confidence of a nation—people could no longer believe the AIDS wildfire would soon be under control. They could no longer accept their leaders reassurances about the cost of fighting that wildfire. The Health Protection Act was repealed, and the neo-segregation ended.

He returned to the podium, then continued. "Ladies and gentlemen, I am that man who was forced to delay his dream of surgical practice. Instead, I became an educator, never to join my HIV-negative colleagues on the front lines of surgical care—never to enter the operating room.

"But all that is the story of one man, you say. You're right, but now I ask you to take a broader view. AIDS is one of the most destructive epidemics in recorded history. Today it is one of the leading causes of death in the entire world. People like you identified AIDS as a disease in 1981. Two years later the Human Immunodeficiency Virus was described as the infectious agent that caused it. Now, more than two decades later, many people in our country still think one of two things about HIV: they either believe it's a death sentence, or they believe it's basically nothing to worry about anymore. Of course, reality lies somewhere between those two extremes.

"People with HIV now live just about as long as everyone else does—provided they start antiviral treatment while their immune systems are still strong. As you know well, there are dozens of different HIV medications, and when the right medications are combined in the right way, they can keep people with HIV healthy indefinitely. But other people, people outside this room, need to know anti-retroviral drugs do not cure HIV infection. The medications do improve the quality of patients' lives, and taking multiple drugs that attack different targets in the virus's life cycle can decrease the body's total burden of HIV. Today's medications do help to maintain immune function and help prevent opportunistic infections that often lead to death."

Jeremy took a drink from the water glass on the podium.

"Do we dare put the words, HIV and cure in the same sentence? I say yes. We can still win the war against HIV. An international push to wipe out polio has yielded stunning results since 1988. Smallpox has been virtually eradicated. If we can get rid of scourges like those, we can surely wind down the incidence of HIV-AIDS. When this epidemic is finally over, and it will be over, two kinds of people will be remembered: those who fought to end it, and those who slowed us down."

He paused for a long moment, then flashed a big smile.

"I have dealt with some of those who slowed us down, but everyone here belongs to the first kind: those who fight to end the epidemic. Together, we must fight on to keep hope alive for the millions who await the successful outcome of our work. Together we must…"

ABOUT THE AUTHOR

George Beddingfield is a physician. Born in Valdosta, Georgia, he attended Emory University and earned his MD degree from Tulane University. He retired from surgical practice and from hospital accreditation surveys for The Joint Commission in 2008 to devote himself full time to fiction writing. He created the basis for *WILDFIRE* in 1990, then put it aside until 2014 when a complete re-write produced this novel. In the interim, he published three additional novels. George lives in San Antonio. Readers are invited to follow the progress of his future works of fiction at www.georgebeddingfield.com. E-mail comments are welcome at gbeddingfield@att.net.

www.ingramcontent.com/pod-product-compliance
Lightning Source LLC
Chambersburg PA
CBHW071401170526
45165CB00001B/131
* 9 7 8 1 5 0 0 9 1 8 0 3 3 *